Chiropractic Works!

ह्ब

Adjusting to a Higher Quality of Life

By Timothy J. Feuling

Wellness Solutions

Chiropractic Works!
Adjusting to a
Higher Quality of Life

Published by: Wellness Solutions

ISBN: 0-9670830-0-1

Library of Congress: 99-93723

Printed in the United State of America
      5 6 7 8 9 10 11 12

Photos of B.J. Palmer and D.D. Palmer used with permission of Palmer College of Chiropractic Archives. Cover photo © David Hiser, Photographers/Aspen, Inc.

DEDICATION

I dedicate this book to every child in the world, for
representing the innocence of life, the beginning of an
unshaped mind, and the future of humanity. Children have
taught me to love unconditionally, to be patient with others and
to question everything to find the answers for myself. Our
children represent the next generation, that will question
modern medicine and seek health care from practitioners
who work with the body, not against the body, and who work
inside out, and not outside in. God bless our children.

Acknowledgements

Special thanks and deep appreciation to:

My loving wife, Brooke, for being my best friend and soul mate, for being the best listener in the world, for always having faith in me, for supporting me in everything I do, and for being such a fun-loving, spiritual, caring friend to me every step of the way.

My mother and father, Kathleen and John, for teaching me how to love unconditionally, exceed my own expectations and for supporting me in all of my efforts.

My brother, Thomas, for teaching me to question the norms and discover the truths for myself.

My mother-in-law and father-in-law, Cindy and Terry for introducing me to a very special path and the "chiropractic lifestyle" I live to this day.

My sister-in-law, Shannon, for always expressing compassion, spirituality and a love for life.

My grandfather, James Herman Feuling, God rest his soul, for investing his time into shaping me into the man I am today.

The entire staff at Chiropractic Leadership Alliance/Total Solutions for teaching me to step out of my comfort zone, surge through my fears and to live and love unconditionally.

Linda Bevel, for always being here for me when I need her and for teaching me the basics.

Marty Marsh, for his commitment and talent in transforming my written work into the book you are about to read.

Every chiropractor and chiropractic patient who sent in the testimonials and case studies to make this book possible.

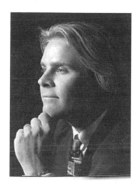

Timothy J. Feuling

Timothy J. Feuling has personally experienced an increased quality of life as a result of years of chiropractic wellness care. While growing up in San Diego, California, Timothy aspired to dedicate his life to helping others discover their inborn potential to excel in both body and mind.

In 1991, Timothy was involved in an accident leaving him with a broken back. Unfamiliar with chiropractic, he was referred around the medical profession, with failed trials of pharmaceuticals and orthopedic recommendations. Orthopedic surgeons were recommending back surgery, but that had to be a last resort as far as Timothy was concerned. A friend recommended chiropractic. Chiropractic significantly enhanced his life, mentally and physically. He was impressed with the quality of care and education he received from his chiropractor. Even more impressive was the enlightenment he was given that chiropractic was not for low back pain, but to allow the "innate" potential of our body's recuperative powers to function at 100%.

Since discovering chiropractic, Timothy's quality of life has improved dramatically, including increased mental acuity, increased energy, consistent relief from the symptoms related to his broken back, loss of stomach problems and head aches and an overall feeling of increased wellness.

While attending Arizona State University, Timothy met Dr. Terry A. Rondberg, President of the World Chiropractic Alliance and author of numerous books and articles about chiropractic care. Timothy started to spend much of his personal time studying the art, philosophy and science of chiropractic, while his work hours were now being spent at the World Chiropractic Alliance. Amazed by the results patients worldwide were experiencing under chiropractic care, Timothy is committed to sharing these powerful chiropractic success stories with the world.

Chiropractic Works! Adjusting to a Higher Quality of Life is one of his contributions to society.

Timothy is Vice President of the World Chiropractic Alliance and Chiropractic Benefit Services Malpractice Insurance Program. He is the co-author of *Chiropractic: Compassion and Expectation,* a book focused on the objectives of chiropractic care and what a patient seeking chiropractic care may expect. Timothy currently speaks to chiropractors and chiropractic students across the nation about compassion and setting expectations. He has recently began arranging chiropractic health care classes for the public in order to reposition the chiropractic paradigm from back pain relief to wellness care and life enhancement.

Foreword

I am not exaggerating when I say this book is one of the most important volumes to be published in recent years and that we all owe a debt of gratitude to its author, Timothy J. Feuling. He has provided us with some of the most inspiring, uplifting, and emotionally moving health stories anyone will ever read.

Feuling has managed to push his way past the obstacles set up by the medical and pharmaceutical industries and defeat their attempt to silence anyone who tries to write or talk about non-allopathic health care choices. The importance of this kind of effort was made clear to me not long after I became a chiropractor.

One of my patients was a young man named George Roberts who, for several years, had been suffering with seizures from epilepsy and was not able to obtain a drivers license because of his condition. He was on very strong medications to try and control his convulsions which often led to unconsciousness. Out of desperation, he followed a friend's advice and decided to try chiropractic.

When I told him that, as a chiropractor, I didn't "treat" epilepsy, he started to get up and leave. I noticed tears in his eyes. "You were my last chance," he said. "Now you're telling me you can't help me either." I asked him to please sit down again and explained, "I didn't say I couldn't help, I only said I didn't diagnose or treat any condition or disease including epilepsy. However, what I can do is examine you to see if you have any vertebral subluxations also known as spinal nerve interference. By eliminating this kind of interference in your nerve system, the master controller of your body, it might allow your own body to heal itself. If there is any interference with nerve function, there will be interference with the ability of the body to heal and regulate itself."

Just getting to my office was a hassle. George had to transfer public buses twice just to reach my office and he did this three times a week. After a few months of care, during which I adjusted his spine and began correcting his subluxations, he told me he never got seizures anymore and was no longer on his medication. "I can't believe it," he said, grinning at me. "I actually feel normal for the first time in my life, I even got my drivers license." then, his smile faded a bit and he shook his head. "But what I really can't understand is why — during all the time I had those miserable seizures — no one ever told me about chiropractic. Not my medical doctors or my pharmacist; no one. None of the things I ever read about epilepsy ever mentioned trying chiropractic care either. That just isn't right."

I agree. It isn't right that news and information about chiropractic has been suppressed for so many years. But it is an undeniable fact that chiropractic poses a threat to the medical monopoly. If people live a chiropractic wellness lifestyle without having to rely on drugs and surgery, except in emergencies, the house of cards built by the medical and drug industries could topple.

That's why the medical establishment and pharmaceutical companies spend millions of dollars every month to get positive news coverage. According to The Wall Street Journal, television reporters rely almost solely on the more than 2,000 "video news releases" sent to them each year by drug makers and medical device makers. Reporters don't ask questions or even attempt to present a balanced report — they simply show the video, which is often little more than a sales pitch for the current "miracle drug."

The same is true for newspapers and magazines. Their articles are usually based on, and often repeated verbatim from, press releases distributed by medical or pharmaceutical concerns. A New York Times article revealed that, according to a survey of 2,500 editors and reporters around the country, 90% of all ideas for health articles had originated with a public relations person representing either a medical or pharmaceutical client!

In addition, the major medical trade organizations like the AMA spend huge amounts of money to ensure that coverage for any competing discipline is either non-existent or — better yet — negative. All of which has left consumers in the dark about what chiropractic care is and what it can do for them. Some of those who are influenced by the millions of dollars spent on medical and pharmaceutical advertising, continue to suffer from poor health, weak immune systems, symptoms and conditions which can negatively affect their quality of life. Unfortunately, many of them end up sicker than they were when they started, as a result of the drugs and procedures they choose to endure. If only they knew...

Now they can know the truth. Thanks to Timothy Feuling's new book, *Chiropractic Works*, people all over the world will have a chance to learn what over 50 million other people around the world already know: chiropractic wellness care will greatly improve the quality of your life, allowing you to function at your highest level resulting in a healthier, and happier life.

Feuling writes with enthusiasm that only comes from the strength of personal conviction. He has done an incredible job compiling these emotionally charged real life stories about real people whose lives were changed for the better as a result of chiropractic care. He shares with us some of the stories of chiropractic regarding actual cases which reflect the health concerns so many of us have experienced in our lives. His love of chiropractic is evident on every page, and he is a shining example of what one person — whose own life was transformed by chiropractic — can do for the world.

— Terry A. Rondberg, D.C.
President, World Chiropractic Alliance

"The doctor of the future will give no medicine, but will interest his patients in the care of the human frame, in diet, and in the cause of the prevention of disease."
— Thomas Edison

THE BIG IDEA

A slip on the snowy sidewalk in winter is a small thing. It happens to millions.

A fall from a ladder in the summer is a small thing. It happens to millions.

The slip or fall produces a subluxation. The subluxation is a small thing.

The subluxation produces pressure on a nerve. That pressure is a small thing.

That decreased flowing produces a dis-eased body and brain. That is a big thing to that man.

Multiply that sick man by a thousand, and you control the physical and mental welfare of a city.

Multiply that man by one hundred thirty million, and you forecast and can prophesy the physical and mental status of a nation.

So the slip or fall, the subluxation, pressure, flow of mental images and dis-ease are big enough to control the thoughts and actions of a nation.

Now comes a man. And one man is a small thing.

This man gives an adjustment. The adjustment is a small thing.

The adjustment replaces the subluxation. That is a small thing.

The adjusted subluxation releases pressure upon nerves. That is a small thing.

The released pressure restores health to a man. This is a big thing to that man.

Multiply that well man by a thousand, and you step up the physical and mental welfare of a city.

Multiply that well man by a million, and you increase the efficiency of a state.

Multiply that well man by a hundred thirty million, and you have produced a healthy, wealthy, and better race for posterity.

So, the adjustment of the subluxation to release pressure upon nerves, to restore mental impulse flow, to restore health, is big enough to rebuild the thoughts and actions of the world.

The idea that knows the cause, that can correct the cause of dis-ease, is one of the biggest ideas known. Without it, nations fall; with it, nations rise.

This idea is the biggest I know of.

— *B.J. Palmer, 1944*

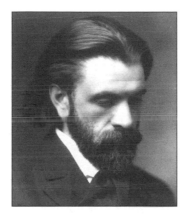

"Chiropractic is a science of the cause of things natural; not a science of symptoms; not a science to chemically analyze the constituents of the human body (normal or abnormal). But it is the science of how to analyze certain conditions quickly back to the cause, and we only utilize conditions in so far as they exist as a guidepost or mile-post on the road, telling us purely which way we must go."

B.J. Palmer
"Developer of Chiropractic"

Why Didn't We Know?
by B. G. Fowler, 1993

A child without his hearing,
Was checked in every way,
By doctors and by specialists,
And this is what they say,

Johnny's going to have a hearing loss,
There's little we can do,
We did a lot of testing,
And checked him through and through,

He may get well with surgery,
And a hearing aids a chance,
Of course there are no guarantees,
And a bank may help finance.

The mom and dad were scared to death,
They knew not what to do,
Should they just accept the fact,
That all these doctor's knew?

A friend of theirs had told them
There is something you can do,
Turn to Chiropractic,
Johnny's hearing may improve.

They took him down to see a man,
Who had practiced many years,
He talked to them and calmed them down,
And looked at Johnny's ears.

The doctor then adjusted him,
At C2 and three and four,
And sent him home to rest awhile,
Then come back soon for more.

The very next day the parents called,
Their voice was filled with fear,
Some blood was on his pillow,
It had come from Johnny's ears.

They brought the boy back in that day,
Quite sure it was a waste,
But Johnny had reacted,
Where their tires screeched in haste.

They knew he had his hearing back
A miracle was achieved,
For all the things they'd been through,
Their stress was now relieved.

They praised the doctor and thanked him,
Their faces all aglow,
He heard them say as they left the room,
"Why didn't we know?"

Why I am a Doctor of Chiropractic

Because I honor the inborn potential of everyone to be truly healthy. Because I desire to help the newborn, the aged, and those without hope. Because I choose to care for the patient with the disease, not the disease. Because I wish to assist rather than intrude; to free rather than control. Because I seek to correct the cause, not its effect. Because I know doctors do not heal, only the body can heal itself. Because I have been called to serve others. Because I want to make a difference. Because everyday I get to witness miracles.

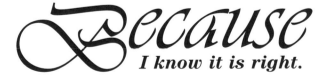

Because I know it is right.

William Esteb
©1992 William Esteb

Chiropractic Works!

C hiropractic patients throughout the world are raving about the incredible results they have experienced while under chiropractic care. Arnold Schwarzenegger recently commented, "I just want to tell you that I am a strong believer in chiropractic because of my first hand experience... There are still people skeptical about it, but they are always skeptical about miracles; it's an advantage when they are a little skeptical, because they say, 'I can't believe that this can make me feel better just like that, without a shot, without drugs...' It is amazing - and that is what is unbelievable for people. I have seen first hand how it works." Arnold Schwarzenegger has been a chiropractic patient for over 20 years. He is just one out of the millions of people that visit a chiropractor on a regular basis.

Over 25 million Americans will visit a chiropractor this year. Chiropractic care is the largest "wellness" profession in the world. When I began to hear of the astounding number of cases of Americans experiencing incredible health benefits under chiropractic care, I made it my responsibility to ensure that these miraculous cases reached the homes of every man, woman and child. I know I can't guarantee this book will reach everyone, but making the information available is my first step in a long journey.

Chiropractic Works! Adjusting to a Higher Quality of Life is a book written with our children in mind. Though the book contains many cases involving men and women of all ages, the cases involving the children are the most incredible. By taking our children to a chiropractor, they will benefit from a system free of nerve interference. Traumatic births, slips and falls, bumping, twisting and sports injuries affect our children day in and day out. The spinal cord and brain of a child is constantly developing over their childhood. These events cause either minor or major traumas to our kids' bodies. We can learn to have their spines checked for nervous system damage.

My goal is to get families to commit to chiropractic care for life time wellness. By bringing our children in for chiropractic care before the traumas have caused permanent nerve damage, we will be acting responsibly as parents. In order to teach our children to take care of their bodies so they will live long, healthy lives, we must set the example for them to follow. This book contains just a small sample of the incredible chiropractic triumphs people throughout the world have experienced. After learning through trial and error within the medical model of "sickness" treatment, these people chose chiropractic care to increase the quality of their life. As a result, the majority of them continue to visit their chiropractor to this day. They have refused to let the medical profession's smear campaign on chiropractic affect their health care choices. Medicine failed where chiropractic succeeded. That was proof enough for them.

The medical profession has discriminated against chiropractic either directly or indirectly ever since chiropractic was discovered. They are opposed to any method of care that is not traditional medicine. It is important to understand their discrimination is purely selfish. The American Medical Association has discriminated against every other type of health care provider. It comes down to one simple reason, money. When Americans visit chiropractors, acupuncturists, homeopaths, naturopaths and massage therapists, they are spending money outside of the medical doctors' offices.

In 1948, the president of the AMA announced they would totally destroy chiropractic by any means. Chiropractic has been under constant attack by the medical profession since its inception. The AMA views chiropractic as a threat to their economy because if people knew they could stay healthier by visiting a chiropractor and having their spines checked for subluxations, they would need less "sickness and disease" treatment from the medical profession. It is a shame so many things in life come down to the almighty dollar, but we have the freedom of choice whether to visit a medical doctor or a chiropractor. The average chiropractic visit costs one half the amount of a visit to a medical doctor.

The United States offers the most expensive medical care in the world. We have the best-trained doctors, more doctors per capita, best-equipped hospitals, leading scientists and researchers, and make more medical discoveries than any other country. This should make us the healthiest nation in the world. However, the practice of medicine is the third leading cause of death in America.

The Journal of the American Medical Association revealed that over 106,000 Americans die annually due to serious adverse drug reactions. Over 180,000 Americans die each year as a result of iatrogenic (doctor caused) injury. Over 150,000 Americans die each year due to medical malpractice. *This is the equivalent of six jumbo jet crashes every week!* Outrageous! In addition to these deaths, approximately 2,216,000 hospitalized patients suffer serious adverse drug reactions.

The treatment of sickness in the United States is a multi-billion dollar business. Millions of people rush into doctors offices every day to treat the symptoms that are plaguing them at the moment. Little do they know that the majority of drugs prescribed have far worse side effects than the symptom they are experiencing. The Children's hospital of Philadelphia reports that nearly three-quarters of all drugs prescribed to children are not approved by the Food and Drug Administration (FDA). In fact, Ritalin has yet to be tested on children under the age of six years old, however, over half a million prescriptions for Ritalin are written for children in this age group each year. Medical doctors are now giving prescriptions over the phone and over the Internet. It should be a crime to prescribe medication without first seeing a patient. However, this occurs on a regular basis. It must stop!

Thanks to the practice of medicine over the years, many of us are convinced that drugs are a harmless thing to take whenever we want to escape from any unpleasant situation. Drugs are often over-prescribed by medical doctors. They do not cure anything, nor will they ever cure anything. They simply make us feel a little more comfortable by masking the symptoms we are experiencing, by depressing the nervous system or by altering our bodily functions so that we don't feel anything.

This is why we take aspirin for a headache on Monday and on Tuesday that same headache returns. We may think we are just getting another headache, but it is the same headache. If a child gets an ear infection one-week and they take antibiotics, the pain and discomfort of the ear infection might disappear for a few days. If the ear infection mysteriously reappears the child is immediately unhappy again. The medication is simply covering up the symptoms and not eliminating the cause of the ear infections.

We need to begin to take responsibility for our health and set better examples for our children in our own households. Our kids learn from our behavior and the examples we set for them. One bad habit we have is running and hiding in a pill bottle or a medicine cabinet every time we experience symptoms or unhappiness. As parents, many of us reach for that bottle of pills every time we get a headache, stomach ache, menstrual cramps, sore throat, cough, have a stressful day, are unhappy, just need a quick pick-me-up or anything that is uncomfortable.

Now, when our kids are growing up, and they are experiencing similar symptoms and stressful events that occur while going through school like bad grades, boy/girl problems, self-esteem problems, etc., it would seem normal for them to take whatever kind of drug they can get to suppress their feelings. Then we wonder why our children do not understand how harmful drugs can be. We have been shaping the minds of our children since they were born. This is why it is so important to set good examples for our children.

The medical profession and the drug companies are to blame for this behavior, since they are the one's promoting and prescribing the medications and convincing us drugs are harmless when prescribed. There is absolutely no such thing as a safe drug. Chiropractors do not prescribe medications and only endorse their use for emergency situations. Chiropractors are opposed to unnecessary medicine. Emergency medicine is a vital part of our public health system, but much of medicine is unnecessary and dangerous. Drugs may make you feel better but not healthier. Drugs can extend the length of the illness by interfering with normal physiology and not allowing the body to heal itself properly.

Chiropractors believe the cause of conditions is a body that is not working right. The body is not able to function normally without a good nerve supply.

We must take responsibility for our health and stop blaming our sickness on external conditions. We get a stomachache and blame it on the food and liquid we ate/drank. We get a headache and blame it on the stress and other outside conditions. We get the flu and blame it on germs and bacteria. This has become an accepted way of reacting to sickness. Our body will heal and improve to its highest level of genetic potential, without nerve interference, and with proper diet, exercise, rest and attitude.

Everyone breathes in the same bacteria and comes in contact with the same germs, but only some of us get sick. Why is this? This is because some of our bodies are healthier and adapt better. Others have bodies that are weak and run down, and are susceptible to the bacteria and germs. We can strive to keep ourselves healthy by eating nutritious foods, exercising regularly, keeping a positive, optimistic attitude, getting lots of rest and visiting our chiropractor on a wellness schedule.

It is important to understand it is not normal for us to get sick, have headaches on a regular basis, feel run down and tired every night, get sore throats and allergic reactions. When we get sick, we need to ask ourselves why our body has failed to keep us healthy. We either believe our body is meant to be sick or it is meant to be healthy. Do we really think we were meant to be sick all of our life? No, of course not. However, we go through our life accepting sickness and disease as normal. We are supposed to be healthy all of our life. Health is built into our body. Our body is supposed to express health all the time.

So, why do we get sick and only concentrate on the symptoms we have at the time? The answer is the drug companies have brainwashed us to believe it is normal to be sick. They want us to believe it is normal to have headaches, feel run down, have sore throats and allergic reactions. Think about how many drug advertisements we are bombarded with everyday, on the television, magazines, newspapers, billboards, radio advertisements, etc. We have been brainwashed to believe it is necessary to take drugs to stay healthy. We should all learn to question the authority of our medical doctors. Ask them why we need a drug, if it will get rid of the cause of our symptoms, condition or disease or just cover up the symptoms, what side effects we might experience and if there are any long-term side effects?

Do not settle for a life of mediocrity! Strive for a life of excellence and health!

The norm seems to be when all else fails, its time to try chiropractic. So many people think chiropractic care may help them, but they are afraid to try it. We need to stop fearing everything except medicine. We should use medicine as a last resort, and visit our chiropractors to maintain our health instead of waiting to treat specific symptoms as they appear. The absence of symptoms does not indicate a state of health. The first sign of heart disease can be a heart attack! Are these people healthy before they get the heart attack and die? Of course not. Chiropractors are trained to restore nerve function to help you become the best you can be. We need to begin to practice wellness.

Chiropractors do not treat disease. They examine the spine to find out if any of the bones are subluxated, interfering with normal function. If there are, they will gently adjust the bones back into position. The body is now capable of restoring the flow of nerve energy throughout the body to every cell, tissue, organ and system, so the body can function better. Chiropractic is based on common sense.

Chiropractic care is solely for the purpose of correcting nerve interference. The body is always striving to heal itself. Nerve interference can be caused by physical, emotional and chemical factors. A subluxation (misalignment) can occur at any level in the spine, causing nerve interference. When these nerves short circuit, the cells, tissues and organs don't receive the proper signal. This results in a state of dis-ease, a "lack of ease" by definition. At this point, symptoms may or may not become present.

As you will discover by reading each of the chiropractic experiences in this book, once nerve interference was corrected, people experienced improved health and their symptoms often disappeared. However, it is important to understand just because symptoms disappear, does not mean we should stop taking good care of ourselves. A good chiropractor will suggest a wellness plan. I believe everyone should visit their chiropractor on a weekly, bi-weekly or monthly basis to have their spine checked. We refer to this as wellness care. As I said before, let's not wait until we get sick to seek care. Let's be proactive. Ask the chiropractor what kind of payment plan is available for your family's spines to be checked on a regular basis.

The chiropractic profession has over 60,000 chiropractors worldwide who are committed to providing gentle chiropractic care. These doctors are dedicated to teach people how to make positive lifestyle changes to minimize the chance of sickness and improve the quality of life.

This book contains personal chiropractic experiences from over one hundred patients, as well as case studies from chiropractors, and a Frequently Asked Questions (FAQ) section in the back of the book to answer many of the most commonly asked questions about chiropractic. Many of the experiences demonstrate how patients exhausted their resources by utilizing medical doctors and pharmaceuticals. They all wish they would have tried chiropractic first.

My purpose in writing this book is to share the knowledge so you can understand and appreciate why Chiropractic Works! By making the choice to begin chiropractic care, you will be taking the first step towards "Adjusting to a higher quality of life."

Enjoy the remarkable chiropractic experiences and case studies presented. When you are finished reading the book, pass it on to a friend so they can understand how effective chiropractic can be.

Who's Who
Under Chiropractic Care

Entertainers

Richard Pryor
"Chiropractic work has helped me a bunch — in ways I didn't imagine. I walk better and I exit buildings better and I think I like myself more. My energy is a whole lot better, too."

Bob Hope
"Chiropractic is a wonderful means of natural healing!"

Dixie Carter, Designing Women TV Series
"I have a wonderful chiropractor. I believe a healthy spine is a healthy body."

Andy Griffith, Matlock TV Series
"Chiropractic has advanced tremendously over the past few decades. It has grown by leaps and bounds to become a specialized and accepted science."

Katherine Kelly Lang, Bold & Beautiful Soap Opera Star
"I leave my chiropractor's office feeling fresh and rejuvenated and back in line the way I should be. He has also been successful at getting rid of my tension headaches."

David Cassidy, The Partridge Family TV Series
(David has been getting adjusted once every three weeks for maintenance care for the last two decades.)
"I've been adjusted so many times that I know when C-7 is out. I know when I need an adjustment. I know what works for me and I trust my own body."

Lou Waters, CNN Today
"I like to go to the chiropractor at least once a week and have for the past 20-25 years. I feel better when I go; I have more energy."

Mel Gibson
He credits chiropractic with helping him keep in top physical form.

Dennis Weaver, "Chester Good" in Gunsmoke TV Series
"It is wonderful to find a chiropractor whose philosophies about healing the body and the mind are in 'sync' with mine."

Brandon Lee, Movie "The Crow"
(Son of Bruce Lee)
He wanted to try chiropractic because he heard it could make the stressful 18 hours of daily filming more tolerable.

Adam Arkin, Chicago Hope
"I have been helped by the healing art of chiropractic throughout most of my life, though I've never suffered any serious chronic health problems.

David Duchovney	**Cher**
Sylvester Stallone	**Jerry Seinfeld**
Robin Williams	**Doris Day**
David Copperfield	**Burt Reynolds**
Denzel Washington	**Robin Wright,** Forest Gump
Whitney Houston	**Meredith Baxter,** Family Ties TV Series
Penny Marshall	**Phyllis Diller**
Kim Bassinger	**James Earl Jones**
Alec Baldwin	**Alan Thicke,** Growing Pains TV Series
Richard Gere	**Patrick Stewart,** Star Trek's Captain
Whoopie Goldberg	Jean-Luc Piccard
Ted Danson	**Clint Eastwood**
Macaulay Culkin	**Linda Hamilton,** Terminator Movies
Demi Moore	**Jane Seymour**
Johnathan Lipnicki	**Dolf Lundgren,** "Rocky IV" Movie
Tea Leoni	**Michael Shurtleff**
Steven Segal	**Heidi Kling**
Dianne Carroll	**Josephine Premice-Fales**
Richard Kuss	**Members of Cosby family**
Johnetta Cole	**David Spade**
Jim & Jan Brolin	

Authors

John Robbins, author of Pulitzer prize-nominated international best seller, "Diet For A New America"
"Chiropractic works in harmony with the basic healing forces of the body, whereas the allopathic, western medical establishment doesn't have nearly as holistic a vision."

Dr. Norman Vincent Peale, Author/Philospher

Candice Pert, Author/Motivational Speaker

Anthony Robbins, Author/Motivational Speaker

Mark Victor Hansen, Author/Motivational Speaker

Fitness Expert

Dr. Joyce Vedral
"Chiropractic helps athletes and people working out, engaging in a sport or even just performing daily functions such as walking and sitting, to operate at their peak levels of performance without pain. I highly recommend that you pay a visit to your local chiropractor."

Recording Artists

Air Supply's Graham Russell
"In my profession as a musician and composer and with a demanding touring schedule, my health and well being are as important to me as my music, and without chiropractic guidance, I would not be able to travel the 100,000 miles every year that I do in perfect health."

Rosanne Cash, Country Singer
She has "sung" the praises of chiropractic. She served as a National Chiropractic Chairperson for the "Stars of Chiropractic" program to spread the word about how great chiropractic is.

Beach Boys

Van Halen	**Members of Grateful Dead**
The Band — Alabama	**Members of Extreme**
Connie Smith	**Members of Bon Jovi**
Travis Tritt	**Members of Dwight Yoakam's Band**
Madonna	**The Eagles**
Kenny Loggins	**Peter Frampton**
Victoria Williams	**Roberta Flack**

Fred Schneider and Kate Pierson — B-52's

Royalty

Princess Diana of England

Sports

A research study conducted by Drs. Anthony Lauro and Brian Mouch, published in the *Journal of Chriropractic Research and*

Clinical Investigation, 1991, indicated chiropractic care might improve athletic performance by as much as 16.7% over a two-week period. The report also concluded that subluxation-free athletes react faster, coordinate better, execute fine movements with improved accuracy and precision, amounting to an overall better athlete

Top Professionals in every sport are under chiropractic care to increase health and performance. The following are just a few sports stars under chiropractic care.

Aerobics

Mindy Mylrea, World Champion
"We put a great deal of stress on our bodies, so chiropractic is very helpful."

Bernard Horn, Mens Champion
"My chiropractor is really phenomenal. He's shown me how to use my body to its greatest advantage. I've gotten stronger and greatly increased my flexibility."

Archery

Larry & Todd Wise, World Champions

Baseball

Jose Canseco, Boston Red Sox
"I've found that it's a great stress reliever to get adjusted. It takes away a lot of the tightness in the muscles, and when calcium deposits form in the neck and lower back, adjustments seem to disperse the deposits."

Wade Boggs, Tampa Bay Devil Rays
"Last year I found Dr. Newman (chiropractor), and I have been seeing him ever since. I have been pain-free and feeling terrific. I swear by it. Now, it is just maintenance and keeping in line so the nerves don't touch."

Greg Mathews, Philadelphia Phillies Pitcher
Credits chiropractic with helping him get off the disabled list and overcome a career-threatening slump.

Ryne Sandberg, Chicago Cubs
His wife Cindy explained, "He's had some awesome games after getting an adjustment. He was frequently adjusted before games."

Mark McGwire, St. Louis Cardinals
John Smoltz, Atlanta Braves
Chris Sabo, Cincinnati Reds
Robby Thompson, San Francisco Giants
Kirt Manwaring, San Francisco Giants
Mark Portugal, San Francisco Giants
Brett Butler, San Francisco Giants
Wes Parker, Los Angeles Dodgers
Don Sutton, Los Angeles Dodgers
Roberto Clemente, Pittsburg Pirates
Rick Monday, Chicago Cubs
Jeff Reardon, New York Mets

Basketball

Dan Schayes, Phoenix Suns
"I use chiropractic as my main source of healthcare. I don't really go to medical doctors unless I need surgery."
Gerald Wilkins, NY Knicks
"I didn't know how much I could improve until I started seeing a chiropractor. Since I've been in chiropractic, I've improved by leaps and bounds, both mentally and physically."
Michael Jordan, Chicago Bulls
Charles Barkley, Houston Rockets
Robert Parish, Boston Celtics
Jack Sikma, Milwaukee Bucks
Scottie Pippin, Chicago Bulls
John Stockton, Utah Jazz

Biathletes

Kenny Sousa
Joel Thompson
Brent Steiner
Fred Klaven

Bodybuilding

Arnold Schwarzenegger, Actor/Bodybuilder
"Bodybuilders and fitness people have been using chiropractors very extensively in order to stay healthy and fit. I found it was better to go to a chiropractor before you get injured. We are a perfect team - the world of fitness and the world of chiropractors."

Dr. Frank Columbo, Actor "Conan the Barbarian" Movies /
   Mr. Olympia, Mr. Universe, Mr. World, Mr. International,
   Mr. Europe, Mr. Italy
Lee Haney, Mr. Olympia (1984–91)
Clifta Coulter, Miss USA
John Defendis, Mr. USA
Grace Lewis, World Champion Powerlifter, Record Holder
Kevin Levrone, Reigning National Champ
Rick Valente, Host of ESPN's "Body Shaping"

Boxing

Evander Holyfield, Heavyweight Champion of the World
"I have to have an adjustment before I go into the ring. It came to the point where I wanted an adjustment everyday. I do believe in chiropractic. I found that going to a chiropractor three times a week helps my performance. The majority of boxers go to get that edge."

Rocky Marciano, Heavyweight Champion, 1956
Jack Dempsey
Tony Lopez
Michael Carbajol
Muhammad Ali

Dancers

Shirley MacLaine
Liza Minnelli
They both call local chiropractors before strenuous shows.
Marcello Angelini
Daniella Buson

Football

Joe Montana, San Francisco 49ers
"I've been seeing a chiropractor and he's really been helping me out a lot. Chiropractic's been a big part of my game."
Joe Montana and 35 of his teammates received chiropractic care right before the 1990 Super Bowl Game.

Irving Fryar, Miami Dolphins
"I definitely believe that chiropractic care has attributed to my fitness. I don't think I could maintain my level of play without chiropractic. When I go to Dr. Napoli for an adjustment I immediately feel better."

Emmett Smith, Dallas Cowboys
"I go see Dr. Bill (chiropractor) when I get bent out of shape on Sundays. Playing in a football game is like being in 30-40 car accidents."

Crawford Kerr, Dallas Cowboys
"Dr. Bill (chiropractor) kept me on the field many times."

Atlanta Falcons Team
San Francisco 49ers Team
Detroit Lions Team
Denver Broncos Team
Dallas Cowboys Team
Ed "Too Tall" Jones, Dallas Cowboys
Charles Haley, Dallas Cowboys
Roger Craig, San Francisco 49ers
Bob Hayes, Dallas Cowboys
Sean Landeta, NY Giants
Paul Fraze, NY Jets Lineman
Ricky Bell
Dammone Johnson
Alex Karras, Detroit Lions
Mark May, Washington Redskins
Gary Clark, Miami Dolphins
Terry Kirby, Miami Dolphins
Keith Jackson, Green Bay Packers
Mike Ingram, Green Bay Packers
Mike Timson, Chicago Bears
Bill Fralic, Atlanta Falcons
Warren Moon, Houston Oilers
Dan Marino, Miami Dolphins
Brian Hansen, New York Jets
Terance Mathis, Atlanta Falcons
Gary Downs, Atlanta Falcons
Byron Hanspard, Atlanta Falcons
Ruffin Hamilton, Atlanta Falcons
Craig Sauer, Atlanta Falcons
Lester Archambeau, Atlanta Falcons
Ronnie Bradford, Atlanta Falcons
Tim Dwight, Atlanta Falcons
Bob Christian, Atlanta Falcons
Joe Profit, Atlanta Falcons
Lenny McGill, Carolina Panthers

Keith Crawford, Kansas City Chiefs
Corey Louchiey, Free Agent

Golfers

Fred Funk, PGA Tour Professional
"I do believe chiropractic has really benefited my game. Over the last three years, I feel I have become more exposed to, and knowledgeable about, the benefits of chiropractic for me and my game. I realize how your body can get out of balance, and chiropractic care helps relieve me."

Barbara Bunkowsky, LPGA Tour Professional
"I have found that chiropractic keeps me flexible and pain-free so that I can perform at my highest level. The benefits of chiropractic have improved my golf swing, putting less stress and strain on my body and allowing me to be a more productive golfer. I believe it also helps prevent other associated injuries that are very common on the LPGA tour."

Tiger Woods	**Donna White**
Patti Rizzo	**Kim Bauer**
Sandra Palmer	**Patty Sheehan**
Lynn Connelly	**Lynn Adams**
Beth Daniel	**Sally Little**
Jan Stephenson	**Amy Alcott**

Gymnastics

Mary Lou Retton
Olga Korbut

Hockey

Detroit Red Wings Team
Wayne Gretzky, Los Angeles Kings
Brett Hall, Dallas Stars

Kick-Boxing

Jorge Angat, Jr., US Lightweight Champion
"The split second that can be added to my speed by my chiropractor could be crucial."

"Chiropractic care gives him that little advantage, that little extra strength and quickness and allows him his best opportunity to regain his title." — Manager - Denis Doucette

Olympic Events

Dan O'Brien, Decathlon
"You obviously can't compete at your fullest if you're not in alignment. And your body can't heal if your back is not in alignment. It was the holistic idea that I liked about chiropractic and that is what track and field is about. Every track and field athlete that I have ever met has seen a chiropractor at one time or another. In track and field, it is absolutely essential. Chiropractic care is one of the things I think that no one has denied or refuted."

Joe Greene, Long Jump
"I know chiropractic helped me. It helped my performance and I feel better."

Donovan Bailey, 100 Meter
Alberto Juantorena, 400 & 800 Meter
Bruce Jenner, Decathalon
Mac Wilkins, Discus
Dwight Stones, Hi-Jump
Edwin Moses, Hurdles
Maria Maricich, Skiing
Suzy Chaffee, Skiing
Mary Decker, Track
Willie Banks, Triple Jump
Joseph Arvay, Wrestler
Nancy Ditz, Marathon

Soccer

Gregg Blasingame, Atlanta Attack Professional Soccer Team
"I was hit into the boards really hard one day and had tremendous back pain. I went to a chiropractor because nothing else was working, and there I found immediate relief."

Brian Haynes, Atlanta Attack Professional Soccer Team
"Chiropractic helps to prevent injuries and speeds up the recovery time when you are injured."

Dr. George Billauer, Team Chiropractor for the
1994 US World Cup Soccer Team
"As the season progressed, virtually every player (had) been adjust-

ed. *Some enjoy it for its preventative approach, and others appreciate the relief it provides them when they have been injured."*

Surfing

Ritchie Rudolph, Professional
"I surfed better than I have in a long time. With just those couple of adjustments, I was noticeably more flexible and had an incredible burst of energy."

Mark Kechele, Professional
"I'm definitely going to make chiropractic part of my training program."

Jeff Booth, Professional
Tennis

Jim Connors
John McEnroe
Ivan Lendl
Billy Jean King
Tracy Austin

Triathletes

Mark Allen
Craig Reynolds
Larry Rhoads

Volleyball

Sinjin Smith
Randy Stoklos
Kent Steffes
Tim Hovland
Craig Moothart
Mary Jo Peppler

Supermodel

Christie Brinkley
"Chiropractic makes me feel a few inches taller each time I come out."

Everyday miracles

Many people have heard the story about how D.D. Palmer "discovered" chiropractic back in 1895. He had a thriving practice in Davenport, Iowa as what was then called a "magnetic" healer. One night, he was working late in his office when the janitor, Harvey Lillard, passed by. The old man was deaf and Palmer was curious as to how he had lost his hearing.

It turns out, Lillard explained, he was picking something up one day when he heard a "pop" in the back of his neck. Almost immediately, he noticed a decrease in his ability to hear and shortly afterwards could barely hear a thing. It had happened years before, and Lillard went to other doctors but finally had given up and accepted the fact he would have to live without sounds.

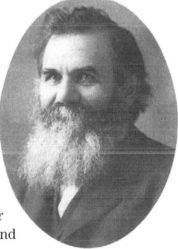

D. D. Palmer
Discovered chiropractic

Palmer pondered the situation. If something "popped" in Lillards neck and made him lose his hearing, could that "something" be popped back so he could hear again? It was an intriguing premise and he began working on the old janitor's neck. He felt for anything that might be "out of place." After a while, he began working the spinal bones in the area, and eventually "adjusted" one of them. Lillard regained his hearing.

That is what got D.D. Palmer interested in learning how the positions of the vertebrae affect nerve function.

This is a similar case of a man whose speech was restored through chiropractic! The case was reported in the Journal of Manipulative and Physiological Therapeutics in 1991 and later summarized in the Health &Wellness report edited by Dean Black, Ph.D.

A 46-year old man suffered from "spasmodic dysphonia," a constriction with the vocal chords that interferes with speech. He went from hoarseness to not being able to speak at all. The condition became so serious that any attempt to talk would make it difficult for him to breathe properly.

After seeing several medical doctors at two university hospitals, he decided to give chiropractic a try. The chiropractor found a vertebral subluxation (misalignment of the vertebra) in his upper spine. After only two adjustments, he was able to speak - although still with some difficulty. After the fifth adjustment, his speech had been completely restored!

It's nice to realize that, had they lived in the same era, these two men — one with new powers of speech and other with restored hearing — would have been able to talk and listen to each other ... thanks to chiropractic.

On August 11, 1990, my 10½ month old son, Jacob, fell off the bed, hit his head and had a stroke. What an utterly devastating experience. He was totally paralyzed on the right side of his body, including his face. His eyes remained open, his face slouched and drool was running out of the right side of his mouth. His breathing was very labored. His right arm and leg were completely motionless.

Chiropractic care began within an hour of the accident. No immediate results were evident, so we rushed to the Children's Hospital where it was confirmed that Jacob had suffered a stroke. We were then given a horrific prognosis: "Your child may never walk, talk, or use his right arm."

Being a chiropractor, and having seen many miracles happen with my patients, I never lost faith, and neither did my wife, Lisa. As frightened as we were, we had confidence that Jacob would come out of it.

I continued to adjust Jacob throughout the night when, finally, approximately 30 hours after the accident, his spine released from the adjustment. Within 30 minutes, Jacob regained full range of motion in his neck and began to move his arm and leg. Two days later, he was alert, smiling and babbling. Ten days later, he was pulling himself up from a laying position to a sitting position. Two months later, he was standing and taking steps. By the end of the year, Jacob was walking.

Jacob is a 9 year old inspiration. He plays basketball, is a red belt in Karate and his mental capacity is 100% plus. While he still maintains some residual weakness in his hand, foot and balance, everyday he achieves new break throughs in his development. Chiropractic remains an integral part of his health, growth and development. Since his accident, we have heard about other children who have had similar accidents and, after years, still remain paralyzed. It scares me to think that, if it were not for chiropractic, Jacob would probably still be paralyzed.

In times of crisis, we all seem to put a lot of faith in medical science and technology. However, if we had listened to the so-called specialists, Jacob would have remained paralyzed. Life is too precious to entrust it solely to medical science. Life is GREATER than science. Thank you chiropractic for turning on the LIFE in Jacob so that he could be well again.

Dr. Eric Plasker, Atlanta, GA

I would like to introduce you to Hannah Rankin. Hannah is a lively and mischievous five year old. If you saw Hannah in the lobby of our office, her brown eyes shining with laughter as she tells the events of the day at school, you would think she was just another pediatric patient coming in for maintenance care. However, her story is a testimony to the power of Chiropractic.

Hannah Rankin was referred to our office on October 29, 1997 when she was four years old. Hannah was having severe problems with her kidneys, as well as suffering from lesser problems like cold type symptoms, general poor health and irritability. She was under the care of doctors at the University of Virginia medical Center, where she was undergoing regular urine analysis and blood work to monitor the steadily decreasing function of her kidneys. Hannah had been on the sodium diet since she was two and a half years old, with little to no success. Hannah's grandmother had suggested her mother bring her in to be checked. Her grandmother had been a patient for nearly a year and was learning about the wonders of Chiropractic.

On their first visit, I explained to Hannah and her mom, Donna, that chiropractic does not treat any specific health problem, but simply increases the body's ability to function by correcting vertebral subluxations. Since subluxation is a big word, we talked about it so Hannah could understand and not be afraid. We then proceeded to check Hannah's spine for subluxations. Her x-rays revealed an Atlas subluxation (listing ASRP), T9 (listing posterior) and S2 segment (listing posterior.) Nervoscope readings indicated severely increased heat at these levels and edema was present as well. The analysis and adjusting technique used was strictly Gonstead. Motion palpation revealed decreased joint motion. We found thermal readings that were extremely high throughout her entire spine.

Hannah's first adjustment was on that same day. Hannah had been shy and apprehensive during the first part of the visit, but became emotional when we went into the adjusting room. Hanna began crying and telling her mom she wanted to leave. Donna explained Hannah had been through so many painful procedures and health problems she was always scared now. Please remember Hannah is only four years old and already associating pain and fear with visits to any doctor. So Hannah and I made a deal, which involved several tootsie rolls, and she received her first Chiropractic adjustment. Hannah immediately became a fan of Chiropractic, because the adjustment had not caused her any pain.

I recommended to Donna that Hannah be seen three times a week for two months then we would reevaluate. Before her first adjustment, Hannah had just been examined at UVA. That examination had revealed Hannah's levels were steadily getting worse. After a few adjustments, Donna began noticing drastic improvements in Hannah's overall health. Hannah was not getting sick, she was able to eat better, she slept better and woke up in better moods. Donna claimed Hannah was a different child.

At the end of the two months, I extended Hannah's care plan to two more weeks at three times a week, two months at two times a week and then six weeks at once a week. During this care plan, Hannah turned five years old and was always excited to come for her adjustment, even at such a young age she recognized what Chiropractic was doing for her.

As spring approached, so did Hannah's regularly scheduled visit and exams at the University of Virginia Medical Center. On April 3, 1998 Hannah and her mom came in to the office with Hannah's results. According to Donna, the medical doctor came into the exam room absolutely puzzled. The doctors explained Hannah's results were perfect, her kidney's were functioning normally. The doctor asked Donna if she was doing anything different for Hannah, and Donna explained she had been taking Hannah to a Chiropractor. The doctor asked Donna if she thought the Chiropractic visits were helping Hannah, and Donna simply replied, "you have the results." At the conclusion of the visit, the doctor told Donna they would not need to see Hannah for another year, and that visit would be just to make sure Hannah's kidneys were still functioning at that level.

Hannah's Chiropractic adjustments were given at the levels of C1, T9 and S2. All three levels were not always adjusted, only those showing signs of subluxation. Hannah's latest thermal scan shows amazing improvements, especially when compared to the original scan. I truly believe Chiropractic changed this little girl's life, but more importantly she believes it and her family believes it. Hannah and her entire family are regular patients who use chiropractic to maintain good health. None of them suffer from back or neck pain, but all of them understand the importance of subluxation correction.

Dr Jim McFadden – Pittsburgh, PA

Seven year-old Becky, had a history of bronchial asthma and bronchitis since she was eight months old. She was unable to laugh, run, play, or bicycle hard without continued coughing, that untreated, led to bronchitis. Between October and March, she would have so many bouts of bronchitis that she was taking Amoxicillin two weeks on and two weeks off. In the summer of 1994, she went to an asthma specialist so she could get off the Amoxicillin. That resulted in weekly allergy injections and two inhalers to be used three times a day. When she got bronchitis again at the end of the summer, another inhaler was prescribed. Perhaps the Amoxicillin was better.

Becky's parents were currently seeing a chiropractor for themselves. Their chiropractor had a wonderful library available for his patients. Becky's mother read about chiropractic care and asthma relief and decided to give it a try for Becky. By December, in a 3-month period, she had not had bronchitis, nor had she had coughing fits. Becky can laugh, run, play, and bicycle unrestricted. She is no longer taking Amoxicillin, or allergy injections, or inhalers. Becky now prefers chiropractic care as opposed to the alternatives. She is now able to live the life she deserves, unrestricted by the limitation asthma used to have on her life.

Becky — Norfolk, Virginia

I had learned about chiropractic after a back injury. Year's later I had a drainage problem in my right ear. I had lost 50% of my hearing in that ear.

When it happened, I went to a M.D. and was prescribed antibiotics. I spent hundreds of dollars on the drugs being prescribed to me. After the antibiotics failed, a tube was inserted into my right eardrum to help the hearing and drainage. Every time I took a shower, I would have to insert earplugs. The tube lasted only 1 year.

Wanting to avoid replacing the ear tube, I mentioned my problem to my chiropractor. I did not expect my chiropractor to tell me he could help. One adjustment in my neck area and my hearing came back instantly! No tubes or pills, just one specific adjustment! Most people take hearing for granted, but when you lose your hearing, life changes. I am so grateful for the life my chiropractor has restored for me. I will never take anything for granted.

Jim — Rock Hill, South Carolina

In a four-month period, Clinton had visited his chiropractor on a regular basis. He came in with such intense pain in his shoulders, that he felt as though he was losing the use of both arms. He was told chiropractic could not remove his ailments, but would allow his body to get stronger and then the recuperative powers of his body would help him feel better.

Clinton had not mentioned quite a few problems he had experienced throughout his life to his chiropractor. However, for the first year ever, he had no allergies or hay fever and was able to avoid taking medication all year. His breathing had improved. He was now taking only 1/2 of the acid reducer, Zantax, he normally required, and was planning on quitting all together. On top of all that, Clinton felt as though he thought clearer and his memory had improved. He knows it is hard to believe all of these improvements came about as a result of regular visits to a chiropractor, but they did.

Clinton's wife, Alice, and his son, Anthony, are also huge fans of chiropractic now. They too have experienced great results.

Clinton — Herndon, Virginia

I had gone to my doctor for a hearing evaluation and was diagnosed with diminished hearing in both ears. Two years later I thought I would try chiropractic. After my second adjustment, I suddenly realized my hearing had greatly improved. I actually felt my ears "open up." "The amazing feeling was similar to when you are a child and have been swimming in a pool all day and you get out and the water suddenly runs out of your ears and full hearing is restored." I was shocked!

That was not the only benefit I had experienced from my chiropractic adjustments. My energy level has increased dramatically. My craving for sugar has decreased and I am now making better dietary choices including more fruits and vegetables and fewer processed foods. The health care classes my chiropractor provides have given me healthy ammunition to make major lifestyle changes. I am still seeing my chiropractor and look forward to working toward total health and well being.

Claudia — Reston, VA

I was introduced to chiropractic by a friend who lives with the same challenge I do: multiple sclerosis. I was hesitant to go see a chiropractor because I was in the midst of an exacerbation of Multiple Sclerosis (MS) that had me mostly numb, the right side of my body dragging, and severe headaches. After attending a local chiropractor's health care class, I agreed to try chiropractic.

I was put on a program where I would be adjusted three times weekly. After just two weeks, I began to notice improvement in my health. The numbness started to subside, and within three more weeks, my body stopped dragging. I was astonished my exacerbation never got any worse. Suddenly, here I was six weeks later with feeling in my extremities, virtually no headaches, and all signs of dragging gone. A miracle!

I continue to see my chiropractor to this day. With a belief in the power of my body to heal and the gentle nurturing of a truly skilled chiropractor, the extent of my MS has been limited to light hand and feet numbness that ceases immediately after adjustment. I cannot possibly express all of the respect and love I hold for my chiropractor and his staff. I am now a firm believer in chiropractic for everybody. I hope anybody with multiple sclerosis will have faith and try chiropractic.

Nancy insisted we include a short list of other improvements she has experienced since visiting her chiropractor. The list includes improved memory, vitality, stamina, body movement, focus, balance, agility, and her eyesight. God Bless!

Nancy – Austin, TX

On July 3, 1994, I began to experience headaches of such a magnitude that there are not words to adequately describe the unbelievably excruciating pain. In the beginning I would experience two-to-three each day, for one week. For the next two and one-half months these headaches were to occur every hour, on the hour, 24 hours a day, seven days a week, and last in duration for 50 minutes.

It was one month after their initial appearance when for the first time in my life I heard the term "cluster headaches," otherwise referred to as "suicide headaches." I was informed this type of headache was very rare, with no known cause or cure. The treatment plan I was to receive centered entirely upon treating the symptom of pain, and not the problem.

With each headache I grew physically weaker, and emotionally more despondent, to the extent of hospitalization. In short, an atmosphere of utter helplessness and hopelessness enclosed around my family like a heavy black blanket. For me, suicide became a serious consideration.

After a few years of experiencing these headaches, they got to be too much. The pain would be so intense I would clench my teeth to the point where six of my teeth split in half. My family doctor referred me to an ENT doctor and he convinced me I needed sinus surgery. As a result of this surgery, I now suffer with permanent loss of all sensation to the left side of my face, while the headaches remain.

By this time, I was totally desperate for relief. Some months before my surgery, my wife and I had attended a health fair in San Diego. A chiropractor was one of the main speakers. Though I had never imagined going to a chiropractor, I felt I had no other choice.

The chiropractor took three X-rays, and within 24 hours was able to determine the culprit was not in my head, nor was it hopeless and without cure. He went on to explain that the top two vertebrae sideslipped and twisted to exert pressure on to the brainstem.

After only three visits with my chiropractor, I can sincerely say the headaches disappeared and I now feel better than I have, or at least can remember, before. I will always try chiropractic first, from this point on.

Jonathan — Carlsbad, CA

I had been experiencing a lot of lower back and abdominal pain for more than a year. My regular physician put me through numerous tests, which were no fun: two kidney IVP Drip tests (the dye they infect you with makes you nauseous), two gall bladder tests, a pelvic ultrasound and an upper GI series. Between the tests and office visits, I was taking Motrin to try and ease the pain.

Since all the tests came back negative (which was good news) there was nothing to explain the pain I still had. The next step for me was to go into the hospital for exploratory surgery.

This is when I decided to call up a chiropractor a friend of mine was seeing on a regular basis. I had never been to a chiropractor before, and I was skeptical, but I was willing to try anything before surgery. This turned out to be the best decision I could have made.

On my first visit, I was speaking with the doctor's C. A. She was getting a brief history from me and we started to discuss how my husband and I never had a child together. We had never used birth control, but I never got pregnant. I had never seen a doctor about why I could not conceive. The C.A. joked about it and said, "maybe the doctor's adjustment would help." Yeah right!

After meeting with the doctor and giving him my history up to that point, he examined my spine and took some X-rays to confirm his suspicion of what the problem was. A few days later, I watched a video about chiropractic care and he explained his findings. After telling me I would feel some pressure but no pain, the doctor gave me my first adjustment. I came to him daily in the beginning and now I visit once or twice a month.

I felt great after my adjustments and after a few weeks, I didn't know why it had taken me so long to find chiropractic. After all the adjustments I have had so far, I feel great, my persistent pain is completely gone, and I did not have to have surgery. I thank my chiropractor with all my heart, not only for correcting my original problem, but also for introducing me to a healthier lifestyle. I especially thank him because I am now the proud mother of two beautiful twin boys. GOD is the only one who knows for sure, but I believe my chiropractor had a lot to do with these births.

Susan — St. Louis, MO

I am a dental hygienist, and my husband and I have been married for eight years. Ever since high school, I had abdominal cramping and pain with my menstrual cycle. For two weeks out of four, I suffered with severe pain. I consulted M.D.s off and on for a year. They recommended a series of GI X-rays and told my husband and I that I couldn't get pregnant. For the last six years of our marriage, we had been trying to have a baby, with no result.

The doctors also said I had endometriosis and recommended I take birth control pills. I did for four months and they did not help. Then, in 1996, I developed neck pain due to leaning over patients all day long in the dental chair. My sister recommended I go see her chiropractor. When the chiropractor took a careful history of my problem, she asked me about my endometriosis and infertility problem. She also took X-rays. She told me there was nerve pressure in my neck and spine and we should begin a series of adjustments to relieve the pressure.

After just a few weeks, my neck pain was completely diminished. Even more miraculous than that, within four months of chiropractic care, I became pregnant. My chiropractor told me I might be able to conceive under chiropractic care, but I had my doubts. For six years my husband and I had been trying to conceive a baby! I really believe the adjustments made it possible for me to become pregnant, and nobody could ever tell me differently.

During my nine-month pregnancy, I was adjusted regularly, and I had a healthy, pain-free pregnancy. Now, my husband and I have our beautiful baby girl, Samantha. Our chiropractor calls Samantha her "chiropractic baby!" She is our pride and joy. We now have the family we always wanted and we have chiropractic.

Joan — Salt Lake City, UT

For the past 10 years, I've suffered from migraine headaches. In the past two years, they've become increasingly more severe and more frequent. I developed neurological complications that affected my right eye and brow. My headaches were completely debilitating at times. It was difficult to function normally at work and at home.

I went to eye doctors, internists, a neurologist, a neuropthamologist, and a headache specialist. I underwent many tests including blood tests, a CAT scan, a MRI, an EEG, an EKG, and an arteriogram. Each doctor prescribed countless drugs. None of the drugs helped, but several caused other reactions.

When I finally went to a chiropractor, I had a severe incapacitating headache for 21 days straight. I was at the end of my rope. I knew nothing about chiropractic, but was willing to try anything.

I finally found some relief! My chiropractor has been caring for me for several months now and my migraines are under control. I have not had a severe headache for quite some time. When I do get a headache, I get adjusted and within an hour I have relief.

I can't say enough good things about chiropractic and recommend it to anyone who wants to feel healthier.

Diane − Sacramento, CA

Deanna was born in March of 1997. She seemed healthy the first day, but by the second she was diagnosed with heart problems. Having to leave her in the hospital while I was released was very difficult. When she was finally released we were so relieved, but little did we know there was much more to come.

At two weeks of age, Deanna had a severe cough and was congested constantly. She was diagnosed with bronchitis. Within two days it got worse and turned into pneumonia and RSV (respiratory syncytial virus). She was again admitted into the hospital.

Even after her release, the congestion continued for over four and one-half months. Deanna was given two kinds of antibiotics, neither one seemed to do any good. She still could not breathe clearly and we were about to the end of our rope.

At this point, we heard about chiropractic. I had never heard about adjusting babies, but we were willing to try. On Deana's very first visit she was very congested, mostly on her right side. She had severe muscle spasms when she was adjusted. Each time we brought Deana back we could notice a difference. She became stronger and stronger in her neck and the congestion seemed to diminish more and more every day.

Her last appointment was August 5 and the congestion is completely gone. Thank God for chiropractic. We now have a baby who was adjusted back to health. Chiropractic Works!

Jim & Gloria – Houston, TX

I am providing this story of regained health through chiropractic. I hope it helps others realize the benefits of chiropractic, because drugs didn't help us. The patients in this story are myself, Tammy Jones, age 26, and my 8-year-old son, Nathan.

I suffered from pain in the back and legs, and simple numbness in the arms and hands. I had this problem since I was 15 years old. I had been to several doctors with no results.

I received a publication from a friend that a local chiropractor distributed to her patients. It discussed various patients who found her work beneficial. I decided I would put her to the test.

In the spring of 1996, I made my first appointment. She thoroughly examined my spine and began to care for me. I got excellent results for my pain and numbness. More importantly, I can now state that 90% of the problems I had from age 15 are gone.

With such extreme results, I asked my chiropractor about my son, Nathan. He had always been a sickly child, but in the past two years it had worsened. He had a constant cough, bronchitis, and more recently pneumonia. There didn't seem to be a time when he was not on one medication or another. None of them seemed to help. Nathan had been on Penicillin for the last two months straight. His medical doctor was about to try and control his symptoms with a steroid, meant for sufferers of asthma.

After his first chiropractic visit, it was determined Nathan had some spinal problems in his upper back. He began getting adjustments and almost immediately I noticed he was not coughing as much in the night. After the third week, he was almost completely free of all coughing. It was amazing to see Nathan regain his health over those few weeks. He had been sick so long and finally he was feeling healthy on a regular basis.

Even know the drugs he used were not working, I never knew there was an alternative for my son and I. I am so thankful for chiropractic. I feel great for the first time in my life and my son's chronic respiratory problems are gone!

Tammy & Nathan — Ft. Lauderdale, FL

My son was born on December 16, 1987. A few hours after his birth we were given devastating news about him. We were told he had a few major problems and they were going to fly him to Children's Hospital in Pittsburgh. He left for the hospital that night. We flew down the next morning. This is when we were informed exactly what was wrong with him. The doctors told us he had a blockage and his kidneys were damaged. He had no function in one kidney and only up to 10% use of the other kidney. His creatine (kidney function) at that time was 4.5. He would need a transplant.

Michael had a few rough months in the beginning. He never even left the hospital until he was five-weeks-old. When we were finally able to take him home, we were supposed to feed him well so he would grow large enough to have a transplant. Michael had what the doctors call reflux. Every time I fed him he threw up the amount in the bottle and more. We couldn't get any weight on him at all. He was born at 10 pounds, 6 ounces and at 10 months he was only 9 pounds.

At the age of four months, he started getting ear infections. He was given antibiotics to rid of them. He would be on the medication for 10 days, off for 2-3 days, and then the ear infections would start all over again. This continued for six months. Finally, the doctor wanted to put tubes in his ears. I did not know what to do. I didn't want him going into the hospital for anymore than we had to. I wanted Michael home with our family.

I was talking with a friend of ours and told her about Michael's problems. She told me I should call her chiropractor and take Michael in for care. I called immediately and they told me I could bring Michael in that day. I explained the whole story about Michael's past and the chiropractor agreed to begin adjusting Michael. He was 10 months old at the time.

After the first adjustment, I noticed a difference. I fed Michael and he kept most of his formula down. We kept going for adjustments three to four times a week and after a month I noticed a lot of improvement. He learned how to sit up alone, he wasn't throwing up as much, he wasn't getting ear infections as often, and his creatine had gone down to 3.0.

Needless to say, we continued taking Michael to get adjusted and after six months of adjustments, he stopped getting ear infections so we didn't have to get the tubes put in his ears. His creatine was fluctuating from 2.0 to 2.7. Quite an improvement!

Getting Michael adjusted bought him some more time to grow

before having his transplant. He received one of his dad's kidneys just three weeks before his third birthday. Since the transplant, he has been doing very well. Michael still gets adjusted about once a week. He has not to this day ever had another ear infection.

Elaine & Michael — Philadelphia, PA

ᘛ•

My daughter, Stacy, now almost five, has had chronic middle ear infections since she was about 18 months old. Each ear infection was hard to treat since the fluid behind her ears would not drain after the infection was gone. She was on antibiotics so much that she began building a resistance to most of them. After awhile, the drugs wouldn't rid of the infections anymore.

Her pediatrician was concerned and told us we were running out of alternatives. Sara might have to have tubes surgically inserted into her ears. As a first-time mom, I couldn't imagine handing my daughter over to a team of surgeons, being put under anesthesia and having surgery.

Our family chiropractor would often suggest that "kids need chiropractic too." I decided to give it a shot. Stacy had just developed another stubborn ear infection, which three sets of antibiotics failed to cure. I could not see her suffer, so I decided to give our trusty chiropractor a try.

After Stacey's first adjustment, on the way out to the car, she said she heard her ears pop and she could hear everything louder. And, guess what?

Her ear infection was gone on her next pediatrician's checkup! Stacy has had a few colds and allergy problems since then, which surely would have caused an ear infection before, but so far she is infection-fee.

I now know that "kids do need chiropractic, too!" What a wonderful, healthy alternative to antibiotics and ear tubes.

Katrina & Stacey — Boston, MA

M y wife, Tina, began chiropractic care following an automobile accident. She responded so well, to our astonishment (since we knew so little about chiropractic) that I began care also.

One day while my wife and I were getting adjustments, we had our 2 1/2 year-old son, Jacob, with us. Our chiropractor noticed he was stuttering. Jacob has a slight speech problem and he sometimes stutters while speaking. He has a hard time getting his words out. We were asked when the problem began, and other questions doctors ask. The doctor thought we might want to have Jacob checked for subluxations, also.

We were skeptical about chiropractic care for Jacob's problem. We just thought it would go away eventually. Well, we decided to give it a try and the results were amazing. Jacob had his first adjustment on August 19 and a few more adjustments in the next week. We noticed between his second and third adjustments he was not stuttering anymore.

Who would have thought a simple adjustment could take away Jacob's stuttering? Our chiropractor is good with Jacob. She makes him relaxed and sort of playful while giving him his adjustment. Jacob can't wait for his next adjustment after he leaves the office each time.

Jacob not only talks better, and we can understand him better, but he has become a much happier child. He gets along with our family much better now. I would recommend everyone try chiropractic. Ever since this event, our whole family gets adjusted on a regular basis.

Our doctor has taught us how the nervous system controls and regulates the whole body, and how a misaligned spine can cause pressure on the spinal cord and cause almost anything. Thank you for great chiropractic care!

Tina, Jeff & Jacob — Missoula, MT

My daughter, who is nine-years-old, has been a bed-wetter since she stopped wearing diapers. I know at her age it is not unusual, but because it was an every night occurrence, I took her to our medical doctor just to make sure there were no infections. She was fine and healthy! Our doctor prescribed medication to try for 10 days. It didn't work at all. So, he prescribed another drug but I could not bring myself to give it to her.

I knew nothing about these drugs and I was concerned with the possible side effects she could experience later. I work for a chiropractor and he explained it could be a subluxation of her lumbar spine. Knowing what I do about the spine and its relationship with nerves, it made sense to me. If a subluxated vertebra is impinging a nerve, the nerve impulse can't travel its path as effectively.

I brought my daughter in and with regular chiropractic adjustments, her bed-wetting decreased. Now, instead of being wet five out of seven days a week, she is dry five out of seven days a week! This has really made life easier on everyone. My daughter is so happy to be dry and I am happy to not have to change bedclothes and sheets so often. It has also given my daughter higher self-esteem. Chiropractic has great benefits to offer children with various problems.

Kristen & Carrie — New York, New York

"Look to the nervous system as the key to maximum health."

— Claudius Galen

For the past two years my 11 year-old son, Timothy, has been a very difficult child. In February, my doctor of chiropractic husband and I attended a chiropractic seminar. We brought Timothy along for the weekend. Timothy had the flu and had to stay in bed most of the time, but he did get to hear a few of the speakers. As Timothy was not well enough to return to school the next week, he had to stay with me at the office, as well as the 25-minute ride each way. I played the chiropractic seminar audiocassettes while we drove and Timothy asked me questions about words he heard.

For the last several years, Timothy had refused to stay still for adjustments. However, after hearing these tapes, he reminded me that "chiropractic is for kids, too," and wanted to start getting adjusted again.

Timothy's health returned with a new attitude to go with it. He started working on his science fair project for school. Timothy chose chiropractic as his project.

He worked hard and wrote about things not commonly related to chiropractic, such as arthritis, asthma, lumbago and the common cold. He also mentioned headaches and whiplash. He then went around his father's office and collected the spines, charts, and pamphlets that he wanted. He made his presentation and this "difficult" child won third place.

Timothy had a realization that chiropractic can help everyone in one way or another. He is right on!

Leslie, Bob & Timothy — Anchorage, AK

I am writing to thank chiropractic for the wonderful results we had lately. My 10 year-old son has been a bed-wetter since he stopped wetting diapers. We had tried seeing medical doctors, pediatricians, and urologists to no avail. My son tried everything from drugs (for five years), exercises, and nasal sprays. We had very little success with drugs, but decided to completely stop taking them because he was just as wet with them as without them.

After four trips to the chiropractor for spinal adjustments, he has stayed dry every night. He is so happy and so are we! I feel so badly when I think of all the shame and sadness he has gone through all of these years. I am so thankful we took the risk to try chiropractic.

There are family members who were skeptical about chiropractic before this miracle that are now not only believers, but also chiropractic patients. They are getting adjusted just for the health purposes.

Brenda — Orange, CT

It was late September 1990 when I was playing high school football and received a very painful injury to my upper and lower back (I pulled the fourth and fifth vertebrae). The impact was so forceful; it took my breath away. I thought I would never be able to play sports again. Then, I was referred to a chiropractor, and it was at this point the tide changed.

He had me list all of my complaints and followed up by asking me to come in for a few visits. In just a few sessions, I saw some progress in my healing process. He then asked me to see him regularly for a week. It was during this time he performed "miracles" with my back. My chiropractor has been adjusting me for about 2 years now, and I am feeling great. I am even able to train and work out on a daily basis again.

My chiropractor even took care of New York Giants star Jim Bunt. When Jim came in to see him, he could barely walk. After receiving chiropractic care, not only was he able to walk again, but he is back on the field playing football. Chiropractic is a gift from GOD!

Brent — Barneveld, NY

On the morning of December 3, 1990, I was two blocks away from work. I stopped at a four-way stop and looked both ways. About 1/8 of a mile away, a car was heading south as I proceeded into the intersection. When he was about 80 feet away, I was thinking he was going to stop. Instead, he plowed into me going about 40 mph, and hit my car broadside.

Wearing my seat belt, my upper body and neck were suddenly stopped because of impact, twisting my upper torso and my neck was jerked resulting in whiplash. All I remembered was my door caving in and suddenly stopping at the intersection

In shock, I got out, took down information and proceeded to work. I ended up taking the rest of the day off so I could go to the doctor and have a check-up.

No X-rays were taken. I was only told to take some Motrin and I could return to work the next day. The next day at work, I was in pain all over my body. My neck, back, and legs really hurt. I made an appointment to see my personal doctor. He did a few tests on me (bending sideways, moving sideways), and then he told me I would never be able to run again. After already finishing four marathons, I was devastated at this news. Running was a huge part of my life.

A friend of mine at work told me to go see a chiropractor. Since I fell into the trap of believing chiropractors were quacks, I didn't take his advice. Three weeks later, in intense pain, I decided to take my friend's advice after all. I made an appointment and as soon as I walked in and explained what had happened, my chiropractor said he could get me running again. How far I could run would depend on me — and on how well my body responded to the adjustments.

I was scheduled for five visits a week for a month, then four visits a week, and then down to three visits a week. After a couple of months, I started walking and jogging to build my back up slowly. I continued a maintenance program to keep myself in training condition.

With the help of my chiropractor and all the trust and understanding he and his staff gave me, I was able to run a marathon again.

In March 1992, I finished the Los Angeles Marathon in 4 hours, 47 minutes, and 17 seconds. I went on to finish another marathon earlier this year. I will be a lifetime chiropractic patient, not only because it helped me run again, but because I feel healthier when I am adjusted regularly.

Sam — Evanston, IL

I am an example of what doctors of chiropractic can do. I was told by my ear doctor that the hole in my right eardrum was getting worse and I would have to have surgery if it continued to enlarge over the next year, when I would have my next check-up.

My mother had been going to a doctor of chiropractic and she had seen a video about what chiropractic could allow the body to do. I started chiropractic care and within just a few visits, the hole in my right eardrum was closed.

My ear doctor could not believe the hole was closed at my next check-up, as I had the hole from the time I first started seeing him at age four - and I am now 25 years-old! You see, chiropractic saved me from having surgery.

I would like to tell everyone, no matter what may be wrong with you, give chiropractic a try and you will feel much better.

Jenny — Little Rock, AR

≈

I am 86 years old. After I had broken my hip and had surgery, the pain in my back and side became very severe. The surgeon said I'd either have to repeat the surgery or rely on pain pills. A M.D. thought exercises would help. She sent me to a physical therapist. After several months I was given a series of exercises to practice. They got so painful; I had to stop doing them.

Then, my daughter took me to her chiropractor. He X-rayed my back and told me I could be helped. He didn't know how long it would take, but if I was willing to try, he could help me. The pain was so severe; I could hardly get out of bed in the morning or up from a chair.

I am a victim of the disease, neurofibromatosis. I have curvature of the spine and unsightly nerve tumors all over my body. Dr. Snyder's treatments have relieved my pain and reduced the tumors.

I started with two visits a week and will soon need to come in only once a month. I wish I had started chiropractic care much sooner. I really was ready to give up. Now, I am a new man.

Ted — Seattle, WA

In 1986, I was involved in a car accident. When I arrived at the hospital, the doctor took a full series of X-rays and found I had pulled all the muscles in my low back and neck. Knowing that, the doctor told me to take a prescription medication and to "take it easy."

A few days later, I called the doctor and asked how long I should continue to take the medication. I was told to continue taking Motrin until the discomfort from the accident had stopped.

In 1988, I was still taking Motrin for my discomfort. Later that year, I started working for a chiropractor. Like many others, I had heard of chiropractic but had never tried it before. During the first few weeks on the job, I saw many patients walking out of the office feeling so good. They would come in with a frown and hop out with a smile.

After seeing the tremendous results other people were having under chiropractic care, I told the doctor about my low back pain and neck pain. After checking my spine, he began adjusting me and I had the same great results all of his other patients had. He was unaware of the stomach problems I had experienced all my life, but the chiropractic adjustments I was getting wiped out that problem on top of the discomfort I had from the accident. Once again chiropractic care performed wonders and I immediately canceled the GI series I had been scheduled for with a medical doctor.

My sister (who also suffered from stomach problems) heard about my success with chiropractic and began getting adjustments, also. She has never felt better!

I learned that problems with the body can often be found and cared for before the person ever experiences symptoms. Many times people think the best way to treat pain and symptoms is to "not treat it at all," so they take medications to cover up their discomfort. That is what I did for 3 years until I learned the power of chiropractic. Now I am drug-free and feeling better than I ever have before. My only regret is I didn't try chiropractic earlier. I could have felt better years ago! Don't make the mistake I did and suffer needlessly.

Susie – Santa Monica, CA

As a young woman of 19, I had my first automobile accident. Twenty-nine days later, I experienced severe pain in my side. The doctors removed a healthy appendix due to negligent diagnosis. In doing so, they discovered I had a ruptured ovary instead, which was repaired.

One year later, I was a passenger in a head-on collision. The injury I sustained appeared superficial - requiring four stitches over the eye and causing a great deal of pain and tenderness in my back. A few days later, I was admitted to the hospital for tests and ultimately, traction. The treatment was pure agony, so I checked myself out and went to a chiropractor.

His care got me back on my feet and the tenderness in my back was eased. Shortly after, I married and had my first child. Once again, another car accident. I began to believe I just had a bad habit of being in the wrong place at the wrong time! My husband and I had no funds, as we were newlyweds with a new child, so I never got any help.

About 15 years and 3 children later, there was another car accident. My passenger and I had not been wearing seatbelts and did sustain injuries. However, the pain wasn't evident until the following day. I began experiencing periodic low back pain, which continued for years, although it was tolerable and I was able to work and maintain a home. Yet this particular pain was different and I began to get frightened.

Although my first thought was to see a chiropractor, my attorney counseled me to seek medical treatment. Believing I should listen to his "professional advice" I placed myself in the hands of a medical doctor. I was given pain medication and placed in traction twice a week for a solid year. What a miserable ordeal that was! The pain became intolerable and there was absolutely no improvement. I now spent hours every day in bed, as fighting the pain was exhausting. Finally, the doctor realized the futility of his treatment and sent me to a neurosurgeon.

The myelogram revealed a herniated L-4 disc, two inches from my spine. It looked like a golf ball had lodged in my back. No wonder I was in such pain. The disc was removed and I spent three weeks in the hospital receiving massive doses of pain medication. It took three more weeks at home to recuperate. The pain was the same but I was told by my doctor, "You will get better, trust me."

About three weeks after returning to work and ingesting painkillers like candy, I could stand pain no longer. Suicide crossed my mind every hour of the day. The neurosurgeon told me to meet him at the hospital immediately for a myelogram - which revealed another herniated disc.

At this point, I was near hysteria. The idea of another operation, the pain, and long recovery devastated me. By now, my physical suffering was beginning to take its toll on my marriage. You might ask, "How did a very strong woman become such a cry-baby?" In response, let me just say unless someone has shared a similar experience, it is impossible to understand the on-going constant pain that radiates down both legs - and the pain trying to rise, walk, or even sit (no comfortable position can be found). There are no words in the English language to adequately describe this kind of relentless, debilitating pain.

The second disc was cut or severed from the nerves, and once again, I went through the pain medication ... and fear. Fear this might not be the final operation. Two years later, the partial disc was removed as it had now herniated. By this time, I was divorced, caring for three teenaged children, and attempting to work. There was more pain, more pain medication, and the constant question on my mind, "Will it ever end?"

I relocated, found employment and tried to go on with my life, all the while experiencing that constant, nagging pain which still extended down my legs and into my lower back. I sought out a doctor for pain medication, and he prescribed Librium. Obviously, he thought the problem was in my head. I threw the prescription back out the door and walked out of his office in tears.

About this time, a fellow employee had an acute infection in her ear and the side of her face from an earring she was allergic to. It was obvious she had a burning infection as her face began to blister. I told her she couldn't ignore it any longer and insisted she go to a doctor. She said, "OK, I'll go to my chiropractor."

"What?" I questioned, "can a chiropractor do?" Yet, after three days of adjustments and massage, the woman's infection was gone! My first reaction was one of complete disbelief. But, it then occurred to me if a chiropractor can help with an infection, maybe — just maybe — he could help me.

I made an appointment with my co-worker's chiropractor that counseled me on nutrition (a foreign word to me at the time), and worked on me for about three months. Each week that went by I experienced a marked improvement. He was able to do something that surgery and pain medication had been unable to accomplish. He explained to me the nerves had been damaged from the surgery and the herniated discs. All he was doing was stimulating the blood flow back to the damaged nerves.

At the end of three months, following years of suffering, the pain was finally GONE! His counseling on nutrition stayed with me as I clearly recognized the benefits. I was now happy, pain-free, and back to my old self.

Fifteen years later and continuing chiropractic maintenance care, it is now hard to believe I went through so much torture for such a long time when it was so unnecessary. Chiropractic care removed the pain and returned me to a normal life. I now work for a chiropractor as a certified chiropractic assistant. I believe sharing my experience with our patients has been beneficial, because I am certainly sympathetic to their complaints and have a good understanding of how to help them.

I have also gone on to learn all I can about proper nutrition. Truly understanding "you are what you eat," I am able to discuss with patients their dietary habits, and advise them if they want to live out their days with quality, medications from a laboratory are not the answer.

I am now 56-years-old and I feel wonderful! I'm very glad I married a younger man — even he has a hard time keeping up with me!

Mary Jo — Los Angeles, CA

ह&

When I started care with a chiropractor, I could not even walk. I shuffled. The first time I came to my chiropractor's office, it took me one hour to travel from my apartment to the seat of my car. The distance I had to travel to get into my car was approximately 100 feet at the most.

I had lower back pain, which traveled around my side and down my leg. I also had cervical pain, which I had been told would need surgery to correct, with a great risk of being paralyzed. My chiropractor helped to correct that situation, also. Some days, I have a little discomfort, but, by and large, I am virtually free of the pain that had prevented me from even holding my grandchildren.

Today, I feel great, can do anything I want to do, using good judgement, and have even returned to my favorite pastime of country dancing. I do all of the other things I enjoy, but could not do for such a long time. I would like to thank my chiropractor and his God-given hands for caring for me.

Theresa — Portland, OR

Just about two years ago, our son fell hard off his bike. He landed right on his buttocks. Some two days later, he started bleeding through the bowels. We went to medical doctors and had all kinds of tests taken. Then they diagnosed ulcerative colitis. We then wondered about the bump injuring the spine, so we went to a chiropractor.

Actually, we saw a total of six different chiropractors, all with different methods. One was helpful in spotting dairy being a factor. The medical doctors said no, but after we demanded the lactose test, we discovered the chiropractor was right. Our son is extremely lactose intolerant.

Another chiropractor got the best control for four days during our son's flare-up. Through many ideas and analyzing, he continued to change the adjustments in a more gradual degree and, at this time, our son is doing quite well. With a combination of chiropractic adjustments twice a month and watching his diet, our son is doing the best he has done since the accident.

The group of chiropractors we chose is a fine group of doctors. We travel 75 miles for an appointment with them over all the other's we've seen. After all the medical doctors and specialists we have been to (including those at the Mayo Clinic), and the thousands of dollars it took to perform and decipher all kinds of tests, it's really amazing this group of chiropractors told us more about our boy's health than all the medical doctors combined.

We only pray in our lifetime we see the day medical doctors open their eyes and help their patients by suggesting chiropractic care. If they would work with chiropractors, what a healthy world this would be.

Patricia, Ward, Dena & Neal — Dayton, OH

Please listen close to this miraculous experience I most recently had with the help of chiropractic care. I would have four-to-five headaches a week. I was suffering from alopecia areata (hair loss) and was experiencing neck pain and difficulty turning my head from side to side.

For my hair loss, I had seen two dermatologists and tried acupuncture with no success. For my headaches, I would take four Advil a day, which only took the pain away and not the headache.

A very close friend of mine that cares for me very much referred me to a local chiropractic office. The chiropractor took X-rays and found my neck and lower back needed work to correct the alignment of my spine. After weeks of care, my headaches have now completely disappeared. My neck is no longer stiff and the best part; my hair is growing back.

I would encourage others, no matter what kind of problems you may have, to try chiropractic. Amazing things may happen like they have for me. Good Luck!

Gloria — Stockton, CA

જ

When I was 8 years old, a group of kids and I were playing and I jumped off a porch. I fell down and hurt myself. From then until I was 10 years old, I limped. All the kids made fun of me, calling me "limpy."

One day I was at a park with my dad. He was playing horseshoes with a man and when I came up to them limping, the man asked my dad what was wrong. My dad told the man how he had taken me to all kinds of doctors and not one was able to help me. The man asked my dad if he would bring me to his chiropractic office and he would see what he could do.

When I went there, he put me on a table and "cracked" me a few times. From then on, I never limped again. The chiropractor would not even let my father pay for the visit. To this day I still visit him on a regular basis to have him check my spine. You should never stop going to a chiropractor.

Jimmy — Mobile, AL

In the beginning, I was experiencing pain in the lower right side of my body, especially my buttock, leg, and knee. I was in so much pain, it was virtually impossible to walk, sit, lie down or perform other than basic functions.

Over a period of time, I progressed through the hands of nine medical doctors. Their diagnosis was diabetic neuropathy. I was afforded a variety of pharmaceuticals and drugs, and a TENS unit, which gave me brief intervals of relief.

During that time, a friend of mine recommended I go see a chiropractor. I talked it over with my wife and she was anxious to see me get well, so she agreed. My wife called to make an appointment and ended up speaking with the chiropractor. She was told I may have a neurological problem and she might be able to help.

The methodology she employed consisted of a variety of adjustive techniques. She told me what her plan of action was and what I might expect over how long a period of time. My chiropractor thought the pain and numbness was from a disc in my spine, and not originating from diabetic neuropathy, as the other doctors had thought. And she was so right!

In the beginning, I told my chiropractor I had very little confidence in chiropractic care, maybe because I didn't know much about it. Like most adults, I did not really have any idea of the importance of the spine or the action of nerves controlling many functions of the body.

I began to improve slowly, but it was remarkable, and to my surprise in line with her timetable. I can hardly believe the pain and suffering completely left me, all without drugs or surgery. The chiropractic care was pleasant and easy, and I now actually look forward to the adjustments.

I not only feel better physically, but also mentally, which was an unexpected bonus. I am regaining my strength gradually, and I am happier overall than I ever figured I could be, at my age. I now advocate if a person begins to feel bad, see a chiropractor FIRST!

Hugh – Portsmouth, NH

I have been working in the medical field for about 20 years. I have always had a lot of faith in doctors, medications, treatments, physical therapy, etc., as this is what I have always dealt with. I have been suffering with a number of different things for the past 10 years. They include panic disorder, heart palpitations, severe and frequent headaches, sinusitis, neck pain, muscle spasms, and one infection after another. I have lost a lot of time at work, per doctors' orders.

The doctors ordered a lot of tests, such as blood work, CAT scans, and MRIs. I saw specialists including a psychologist and a neurologist. They told me I was suffering from severe depression and put me on anti-depressants. They said I was suffering from a panic disorder and they put me on tranquilizers. The neck pain and muscle spasms were treated with anti-inflammatories and muscle relaxants. They said I had cervical arthritis and to take anti-inflammatories for that as well. My doctor got to know me so well that when I got a flare-up of sinusitis, all I had to do was call the office and they'd call me in a prescription for an antibiotic.

I work at a nursing home, on a long term care unit with very difficult patients. I re-injured my neck several times this last year, which led to more time off from work, muscle relaxants and anti-inflammatories. I had physical therapy done for 10 weeks and was on light duty for two months as well.

Then ... the pain came back! I could not move my head either way. I had spasms in both my shoulders which caused them to stay upwards towards my ears. I could not take it anymore!

In July, the director of nursing and a secretary both said to me, "I know what you are going through ... have you thought of seeing a chiropractor?" I said, "Why not? I've tried everything else."

So, I made an appointment with a chiropractor, and I have been under chiropractic care ever since. I learned I had several subluxations which were causing my spasms and pain. All the doctors and the physical therapists had been doing was treating my symptoms - not the problem.

I had two colds recently, and for the first time in six years I did not need antibiotics! My immune system was obviously working again. I have not had a severe headache in months and my panic attacks have lessened in severity. I have also made a huge decrease in my medication. I sleep better, have missed no time from work in 5 months and most importantly I have a better outlook on life itself. I know I still have a long way to go, but I feel I am halfway there and owe thanks to my friends at the Northside Nursing Facility for suggesting I go to a chiropractor.

I now know chiropractic care is not just for back pain, but it is for total health care. If more people would come to realize this, I feel we would have a much healthier, drug-free and pain-free world.

Kendra — Taylorsville, NC

ॐ

For 10 years I suffered from severe pain at the base of my spine. I spoke to several doctors about this and got no results. Finally, I visited a chiropractor who took X-rays and discovered I had a coxic which was turned over on itself three times. This was probably the result of an accident I had been involved in years ago. Within about three months of adjustments, the pain was gone.

During the spring, I developed severe pain in my right shoulder. A few months later, I went back to the chiropractor. He discovered I had disintegrating discs in the spinal column and spurs growing into the nerve.

I began a program of care immediately and within a few months I was able to schedule visits once a month instead of every day and every-other-day as had been the case for the last few months.

During this period, I had also visited my internist, who sent for a CAT scan and a MRI. These tests revealed the same conditions my doctor of chiropractic had discovered, but I was told by the MD there was no treatment except surgery. Thankfully, due to cardiovascular problems, surgery was not an option anyway. Thanks to chiropractic, at this time I am pain-free and can function normally. I now live a much happier life because of my chiropractor.

Dale — Seattle, WA

I had excruciating pain in my right arm and hand for three weeks before consulting a chiropractor. I was unable to sleep or properly care for my family because of the pain. The chiropractor examined me and determined the problem was coming from a pinched nerve in my neck. He told me he would set up a series of adjustments for me. The care he gave was pain-free and I felt better after the first visit.

I was really surprised when I was able to sleep the night through without being awakened by pain. The next morning was equally surprising because my arm felt much better. I was told I was lucky to have such quick results since I had waited so long to seek care. I have chosen to continue care to correct my postural problems so the pain does not return but right now I am happy to be pain-free. I have told my neighbor to see my chiropractor for her back pain as I am sure he can help her also.

Maria — Baltimore, MD

❧

Twenty years ago, I was in a moped accident and broke my big toe. It doesn't sound like much, but it threw my walk off to the extent that over the years I have had various aches and pains on my right side — ankle, knee, hip, and lower back. I have also had shoulder and neck discomfort. I thought it was just old age.

After receiving chiropractic care for 15 months, all of these areas are improved or completely better. I have feeling in my big toe, and can move it now. I walk differently, stand straighter, and am fatigued far less. I seem to be able to handle the stress of life better and think about things more clearly.

I have not been sick in over a year. I have much more energy than I used to and feel more productive in my life. I feel better now at 49 years old than when I was younger.

Alice — Maui, HI

My son, Kenny, who had 50% hearing loss since at least age four and couldn't speak too well, had constant ear infections and fluid in his ears. He was on all different kinds of antibiotics, decongestants, and ear drops. For six-to-eight months we saw one doctor every 10 days.

Finally, we decided to see an ear, nose and throat doctor (a specialist!) who said Kenny needed drainage tubes in his ears to allow fluid to drain. He also advised us to let him take out Kenny's adenoids. He felt they were enlarged and not allowing the fluid to drain. Kenny still got ear infections after the tubes were put in, although not as many. However, less ear infections were not because of the surgery, but because he was no longer allowed to get water in his ears.

After his third set of tubes, I was at the end of my rope. It was then I started seeing a chiropractor for pain in my shoulder (my M.D. couldn't find anything wrong with me or a reason for my pain). While in my chiropractor's office one day, I picked up a few brochures on chiropractic and children with chronic ear problems. I was so tired of running to doctors with Kenny and putting him through the pain of being poked at. The hospital stays were just too much for him and me.

I decided to give my chiropractor a shot with Kenny. A year-and-a-half later, Kenny has not had any ear infections. He does not cry anymore because of ear pain and he can hear everything I say.

I wish I had known about chiropractic when Kenny was four years old. I could have saved him all of the pain and troubles he had to go through. It is so painful for me, as a parent, to watch my child go through surgery 3 times.

As for myself, after about six weeks of chiropractic care, I no longer suffered from shoulder pain. My whole family is healthier because of chiropractic care. We have been taught the importance of chiropractic and will be patients for life.

Theresa - Newark, NJ

In 1989, I was a senior in high school. I had been a swimmer/water-polo player since I was in kindergarten. Therefore, I had always considered myself to be a well-trained and conditioned athlete, free from injury. As my senior year progressed, I started experiencing pain in my lower back. Soon, it progressed into shooting pains down my right leg. The sleepless nights, the unbearable pain, and immobile days told me I had to do something.

At first, aspirin seemed to kill the pain but then I found myself taking an average of six-to-seven a day. This was not healthy and I knew it. Finally, I was referred to a chiropractor in the area.

After meeting her and discussing her holistic approach to chiropractic care, I decided to put my back into her hands. I was still in a lot of pain, but as my chiropractor taught me, chiropractic was not a quick cure, but a lifelong choice for high maintenance.

After two intense months of chiropractic care, daily stretches, and a basic change in my daily behavior, the pain was gone. As a five-year veteran patient, I must say the philosophies and holistic approaches of chiropractic care have influenced and changed my life tremendously.

I enjoy my life on a new level of fitness, a level which allows positive life force to influence my entire body, mind and daily life! I'm a chiropractic patient for life.

Steven — Huntington Beach, CA

ಕ

I wish to thank chiropractic from the bottom of my heart for helping my boy walk again. Joey had been in bed for almost two weeks as his medical doctor prescribed. Joey nor I saw any improvement. He kept placing one shoe on his foot so he could be even. He kept looking in the mirror and wondering if he would ever walk straight again.

Thank GOD for my daughter-in-law, Mary, who recommended her chiropractor could possibly help Joey. I cannot begin to tell everyone how kind my chiropractor was. He would call to see if Joey was O.K. Most doctors today would not take the time to be so considerate.

I appreciate what chiropractic has done for my son. Yes, it does seem like a miracle, when you see someone who has become so deformed stand tall again. You have to believe in miracles, and that's something that money can't buy.

Rudy — Colorado Springs, CO

For about four years, I had been experiencing difficulty in swallowing. Knowing my father had cancer of the esophagus, I was concerned for my health. Medical doctors did tests and took X-rays and identified the problem as constriction of the esophagus, but nothing more was done to help me.

The swallowing difficulty progressively worsened, so I saw a specialist who also tested and X-rayed; then surgical testing - to no avail. He could see the problem but offered no solution. He was just thankful my husband knew the Heimlich maneuver.

Even after all of this, I was having some terrible experiences where I couldn't swallow at all until I waited for what felt like a muscle spasm to relax. A few stressful times, it went on for three days. A new doctor prescribed drugs which I never used.

The real miracle came in the way of chiropractic care. I never would have thought about chiropractic, but it was my last hope. After only 2 months and 15 adjustments, the chiropractic healed me. Now that the neck (C2 and C5) is properly aligned, the muscle can be strengthened. I am no longer experiencing the problems the medical doctors had no solution for. Chiropractic works!

Joan — Eerie, PA

ॐ

I originally went to a chiropractor for pain in my lower back, stemming from a ski injury in 1969. Over the years, the injury has worsened to the point where I am often in severe pain. I decided to visit the chiropractor and give him a crack at it.

This was the most wonderful choice I have ever made. I now have greater flexibility and movement, and removal of the severe pain I have experienced for the last 15 years.

My chiropractor discovered my cervical spine was similar to a "goose neck." Well, in the months that have passed, we have straightened that out. I am now a half-inch taller! My chest has been expanding to the point where I have thrown all of my medium shirts out and replaced them with large shirts to fit my now fuller 6'3" frame.

I am happier, healthier and encourage others to seek the care of a chiropractor. I am now able to hit the slopes again.

Joshua — Denver, CO

Chiropractic has made good sense to me for a long time. I first heard about the "how" and "why" in San Diego, California around 1968 or so. I injured my back when my wife, Susan and I, were helping another couple move. Instead of going to the hospital with the possibility of traction and a lot of pain and discomfort, Susan took me to a chiropractor.

Having been a believer in chiropractic since then, I have pretty much heard most of the "claims," "revelations" and "cures" that surround chiropractic practice. I also understand chiropractic is not necessarily a quick fix. If one gives it a chance to work, it works. I am healthier as a result of chiropractic care.

Recently, when I went to see my chiropractor, a personal experience in his office just blew me away! My hearing was restored! Now, I know that must really sound crazy to anyone who reads this, but it is true!

Due to a draining problem in my right ear, 50% of my hearing in that ear had disappeared years ago. When this happened years ago, I had to spend a lot of cash on doctor visits, antibiotics and then a tube insertion. The tube was inserted for drainage. The tube lasted a year with me having to insert an ear plug every time I took a shower. Not a very fun experience.

Anyway, facing the possibility of another tube in my ear, I mentioned the problem to my chiropractor, not really expecting anything in return. One little adjustment in my neck area and voila! My hearing came back instantly! No tubes, pills, needles or drugs.

When I told my ear specialist what my chiropractor had done, he seemed to understand exactly what had happened. He even gave me the medical names for the bones my chiropractor adjusted.

That raises an interesting question. Why didn't he refer me to a chiropractor? Instead he stuck a tube in my ear, which took a year to heal. I will never know the answer, but I do know chiropractic has been good to me and I recommend it to any and everyone.

Thomas – Spartanburg, SC

When Heather was born, she was a normal, healthy baby. Or so I thought. One morning, before she was two years old, she awoke and came into my bedroom. When I looked into her face, to my shock I saw her eyes were crossed! She had developed a lazy eye on the left side. She is now six and though we have tried patches, exercises and special glasses, nothing seems to make much of a difference.

A few months back, Heather and I were involved in a car accident in which we were rear ended by another car. We were hit so hard my windshield was cracked and my engine was pushed into the radiator. Though Heather didn't complain of any pain in particular, I noticed a marked change in her attitude. She was irritable and quick to anger. She just wasn't my little girl anymore.

After a few weeks of medical care, many pain pills and muscle relaxants plus physical therapy, I just wasn't getting any better so I sought the care of a chiropractor. When I told him about Heather's change in attitude since the accident, he told me to bring her in and he'd check her out. He used his diagnostic equipment and found she had subluxations and she needed to have them corrected.

A few weeks later I had my little girl back! What are even more incredible are Heather's eyes. While her left eye was crossed over 80% of the time before we started care, after only eight weeks of care her eyes are straight at least 80% of the time now! All the time and money spent on the treatment of her eyes only to discover she could heal herself when the subluxations were gone.

Carly (Heather's mother) — Portland, OR

I'm a nurse and I work in a busy Intensive Care Unit. Despite training in body mechanics, the strain of continually lifting and pulling patients started to take its toll on my back. I was having shooting pains down my left leg with numbness in my toes. I had seen other nurses go through physical therapy, take drugs and try to live with chronic back pain. I thought there must be a better way.

A friend suggested a chiropractor. I was skeptical at first but after two adjustments my pain and numbness were gone. Learning more about chiropractic, it just seemed to make good sense. My nurse's training taught me the innervation of the body comes from the spinal cord. The nerves must all pass through the vertebrae to reach organs and tissues. If the vertebrae are out of alignment, this will create pressure on the nerves and produce pain or lessen the function of the organs.

Chiropractic realigns the vertebrae and helps to relieve the pressure. No drugs, no months of physical therapy, and no learning to live with chronic pain. Through regular adjustments, I have been free of pain and I feel great!

Robert — Newark, NJ

ελ

I have had trouble for many months trying to eat and swallow. A spasm of the tongue is what I assume you would call it. When I was upset or went to eat or drink fluid I had trouble. I was on different medications but got no relief: if anything, I got worse. There was just no let up, just a constant ache, day and night. Sometimes when eating I had a coughing spell and would have to wait until it subsided before I could continue eating and take very small amounts of food in my mouth because I couldn't swallow. My throat and ear ached just to touch.

My son was telling me about going to a very good chiropractor and how he was being helped, so I thought maybe he could do something for me. So, I made an appointment.

I'm very happy I went to a chiropractor, for now I am getting relief which did not come from all of the medications. I no longer suffer from all of the side effects of the medications I was taking. I can now sleep on either my right or left side, which I couldn't do before. In other words, I can eat, sleep, drink and be merry thanks to chiropractic.

Doreen — Wichita, KS

J ust a few months ago, I began to experience pressure and numbness in my head. I kept telling myself it was just nerves, hoping it
would go away, but one day the numbness spread to one side of
my face. It really scared me, as it seemed to be warnings of a stroke. I
knew I needed help, but where?

Now, whenever I'm upset or confused, the first thing I do is to plug
into a higher power. As I was praying, I knew in my heart the Lord
would send me to the right doctor. Well, after my first visit with a chiropractor, I knew I had made the right decision. I found my chiropractor to be a man of great faith, and most of all, positive and caring. He
took the time to answer questions and discuss any concerns I had.

After only a few weeks of adjustments, the numbness is completely gone. I am able to go about my daily duties without the fear of having a stroke, and that in and of itself is peace of mind. I thank GOD
every day for the gift of health and for my chiropractor and his instrument of healing!

Brooke — Eugene, OR

M y experience with chiropractic and this office has been
extremely pleasant, educational and rewarding. When I first
came in to the office, I was in a lot of pain. My neck and
shoulder hurt and my left arm and hand were often numb and weak.
Three months later, I feel great!

I have no pain whatsoever. My hand and arm are not weak or
tingly and I can honestly say I have never felt better in my life. Every
winter I get at least 3 sinus infections with terrible headaches. Since
November, when I came in, I have not had one headache or sinus
infection! We have had numerous fires in our fireplace, which are
known to aggravate sinus conditions, and I feel just fine.

Going to a chiropractor was one of the best things I have ever
done. Everyone in the office is so pleasant. I really look forward to
my appointments. When I first came in, my chiropractor said he
would like my adjustments to be the "highlight of my day," and sure
enough - it is!

Nathan — Edgartown, MA

I sure am going to express my honest feeling and experience with chiropractic care. It has helped me tremendously. After many years of frustration, pain and agony, I was not happy or satisfied with my physical condition and did not want to carry on any further. I decided that I should see a chiropractor. I saw a big change in a short period of time. In the meantime, to add insult to injury, I had a terrible home accident. I landed myself in the hospital for ten days with back and hip observation. Many tests were performed (X-rays, MRI's, diets, etc.). They were unable to find anything wrong.

This was the climax. I was determined to change doctors without hesitation and I did just that. When I explained to my chiropractor what had occurred, he said he could help me. Due to a double injury, it would take a little longer. Well, I complied with extensive adjustments and cooperation on my part, and we succeeded!

Yes, many days went by thinking I would not regain my own self-strength, after all, I am 73 years young. I will continue chiropractic care because I have faith in my chiropractor and his teachings.

Lawrence — Redondo Beach, CA

I want to take this time to thank my chiropractor for the wonderful care given to my family and encourage others to begin chiropractic care. Before we came to you, the kids had colds all of the time. They also had other problems, like Billy's asthma, Jake's ear infections and Bobby's bed wetting.

Since we have been under chiropractic care, the kids have never been healthier. Billy's asthma has almost completely subsided. He hasn't had a bout in months. Jake's ear infections are far less common, and Bobby has completely stopped wetting the bed.

I just want everyone to know how much we appreciate and recommend the effectiveness of chiropractic care. I have been recommending chiropractic to all of my co-workers and friends.

The Cornwell Family — Detroit, MI

This letter was written from a chiropractic patient to the parent of a child with chronic asthma.

I have been a chiropractic patient for a couple of years now. I sought chiropractic care for several problems. In passing conversation, my chiropractor told me your son suffers from chronic asthma and is controlling this condition with medication. This has been bothering me for over a week and a half now, so I felt I should write you this letter.

I was afflicted at the age of 6 with chronic asthma, hay fever, a stomach disorder and severe allergies. I was unable to play any sports without medication. I was unable to eat many foods such as pizza, chocolate, ice cream and peanut butter. I was allergic to molds, grass, weeds, pollen, wool and rubber products.

I had been receiving medication, oral and by injection mostly, from 6 to 18 years of age. I then refused all medical treatment for several reasons; unbearable side effects and I couldn't afford the astronomical medical bills. The severe rashes, which occasionally resurface were caused by large doses of medication doctors said were safe. From this I became allergic to pennccillan and all of its derivatives.

Then a few years later, my mom spoke to a woman who was taking her son to a chiropractor for allergy treatment and recommended him to me. I first researched chiropractic and felt good about it helping me with my conditions.

After a few weeks of care, I feel better than I had in 27 years. I no longer take any medication for my allergies or my asthma. I still continue a maintenance program to stay healthy.

I cannot promise a chiropractor will be able to help your son, but if he does, maybe next time 'your' son will be writing this letter to someone who was ill with similar conditions.

I wish you both a life of wellness.

Jonathon — Palm Beach, FL

I originally began chiropractic adjustments to increase my flexibility/mobility. As I received regular, periodic adjustments, I began to notice my overall energy levels and health gradually increase.

Now I come for weekly adjustments because it is a positive thing that I can do to overcome the many stresses of modern life, and it is a way that I can take control of my own health and well-being.

John — Rapid City, SD

෨

Through the torso
Runs a channel
Dense and solid / Slim and fragile;
Balance lends omnipotence
To keep us running
Powerful / Yet agile.

Through the office
Runs the healer
Rushed and mobile / Still in blessing;
Measured by his ink-crowned child
To keep things running
Structured / Yet unstressing.

Through the meadow
Run my children
Open, leaping / Creeping, stealthy
Running in omnipotence
To keep me balanced
As you keep us / Healthy

L.S. Cohen

I can't begin to tell you what chiropractic care has done for me from the preventative maintenance standpoint. I have had less sickness in the past 5 years I have been under chiropractic care than I have ever had in my lifetime. I have improved output since my stress-filled lifestyle has been amended with a weekly — sometimes bi-weekly adjustment. Thanks for helping me experience the Power of Chiropractic.

Alicia — Weed, CA

ed.

I sought chiropractic care at the urging of a friend after I was in a car accident. Although the seatbelt did save my life, I was left with back and neck problems. I underwent 6 weeks of treatment through my medical doctor but still experienced discomfort and sickness. Also, other medical problems began to occur.

I believe in chiropractic because after only a few adjustments, I was pain-free. The stiffness lessened and I was "less afraid" to bend and move in and out of cars. Chiropractic has taught me to look at my whole body: the spiritual, the mental, and the physical. I can see the interconnectiveness of all these components in my life. I've become more attuned to my body and its needs. After always being prone to colds, sinus problems and respiratory problems, I've experienced a new "wellness."

Although not all of my problems have disappeared completely, I've learned through my new awareness to catch them early and the seriousness and the duration of them has lessened. Chiropractic has taught me to work "with" my body....to listen to it....and to enjoy all I can do now.

Sister Denise — Philadelphia, PA

ed.

I started chiropractic care in November, 1986 because of shoulder and neck stiffness. I continue to go once a week. My whole body feels better. If I get colds, they don't last as long. My blood pressure is the best it's ever been. With the adjustments I have much better posture and I don't feel as tired out as I used to.

Mary Ann — Morrisville, PA

My health has improved so dramatically. Friends comment on my walking and posture. My hip retains it's proper positioning. The chiropractic adjustments have enabled me to proceed with my healing schedule, which was not a small undertaking.

After nearly fifteen years of forced retirement from nursing, I am now able to think of returning to my chosen profession. Occasionally, someone who has not seen me for some time is surprised to see me walking so well.

I thank chiropractic so much for my renewed enjoyment of life.

Renee – Oceanside, CA

૨ઃ

Several months ago, I was hospitalized for a stomach ulcer. When I recovered from this illness, I was experiencing fatigue, headaches, and pains in my back and neck due to some former injuries in my life.

I began to pray for God's Wisdom in where I must seek help and then it happened! I met a chiropractor in church and in my heart, I knew this Doctor of Chiropractic would be the one God had brought to my mind.

My chiropractor has been an answer to my prayer; he not only is a fine chiropractor but a very sensitive and caring person who intently desires to help people feel well and think well — a man of great faith in God who prays for his patients. There is a very positive atmosphere in his office which has a definite influence on his patients.

I highly recommend chiropractic care as I can witness to the change in the way I feel. This method of adjustment to the spine where power and healing flows to the other areas of the body is most beneficial to everyone.

May God continue to bless chiropractors and patients day after day to the Praise of Glory of God!

Mary – Philadelphia, PA

A s a runner, jogger and walker, I was experiencing lots of low back distress, as well as sciatica. At the age of 35, the pain was becoming chronic.

A friend who is a medical doctor (a general practitioner) recommended chiropractic care. He exercised regularly and felt chiropractic care was the most effective and most appropriate care for the stress on the body and the spine.

The pain eased immediately. In one month and eight chiropractic adjustments, the pain had vanished. I even noticed my breathing was easier. I was able to sustain longer work-outs and I even slept better. Generally, my health improved in all areas.

I believe in Chiropractic because it works for me. I'm adjusted once a week for a maintenance program. With all of the confidence I approach Chiropractic. Five years ago, two doctors told me to stop running or jogging because of my low back pain. Chiropractic care enabled me to continue and maintain good health. I can now enjoy all kinds of physical exercise.

John — Montgomery, AL

&

I nitially, I came into my chiropractor with a pain in my shoulders, neck and arm. It was the day before my birthday and I saw a chiropractic office on my way home. I had been suffering for some time and after seeing a specialist who prescribed cortizone shots, acupuncture, and pain killers (muscle relaxers - valium), nothing helped me.

I was desperate. I drove into the chiropractic office parking lot, figuring I had nothing to lose. I can't begin to tell you the relief I have gotten from the adjustments I have received!

I couldn't sleep on my side for years without constant pain! Sometimes the tingling and numbness in my hand, arm and shoulder was so bad it would wake me up.

Today, one year later, the pain is completely gone! I can sleep on either side without pain. I still continue to receive chiropractic care because I don't ever want to experience that kind of pain again. I believe with all of my heart that a wellness program without drugs is the only way to a healthier life, and I am living proof!

Anne — Lake Tahoe, NV

I first sought chiropractic care for the treatment of leg and back pain and some tightness in my neck area. My son, who sees a chiropractor regularly, recommended it.

In time, my problems were corrected. I began to feel good; I had much more energy and pep. I accomplish a lot more than I used to and I feel great.

My belief in chiropractic stems from the fact that I feel better than I ever have before — as long as I keep up and get my adjustments regularly, I function better. I have recommended chiropractic care to many people because it works!

Anne — Levittown, PA

My original complaint was shoulder pain that I had for a long time and tried to ignore. The pain bothered me so much I could not sleep on my shoulder. My husband has been going to a chiropractor and kept urging me to make an appointment. I started going to the chiropractor about a year ago.

After many adjustments, I can honestly say my shoulder pain is gone. While going to my chiropractor, he educated me so much through pamphlets, videos, and lectures about chiropractic care. I realized chiropractic care is not only for bodily pain, but for maintaining good health as well.

As a result of this care and knowledge, my whole family now makes weekly visits to our chiropractor to ensure good health.

Pam — Atlanta, GA

Preventative maintenance is a key to ensuring a high level of health. With Chiropractic adjustments, my body is receiving the care it needs along with exercise, good nutrition, etc.

I'm blessed to have good health and don't see any particular changes that stand out. However, knowing I am in proper alignment helps me to feel secure in my all-around quest for health.

As I get older, my level of health remains the same. I believe in chiropractic because I am proof it works.

Bob — Spartanburg, SC

M y initial introduction to chiropractic was an oral report from a high school classmate. Removing interference for a free-flowing nerve supply MADE COMMON SENSE! At the time I was looking for help with severe wrist pain. I could not lift my coffee mug without excruciating pain.

X-rays and doctors' exams proved futile, but chiropractic did the trick for me. After a short time I could lift the coffee cup. After several years I was again able to lift my body during exercise.

I've been under chiropractic care for 15 years. It's a necessary part of my health regime and as habitual now as brushing my teeth. Just as we need to brush our teeth regularly for good oral hygiene, we need to adjust our subluxated vertabrae regularly to maintain a good nerve supply to all the organs in our body. I thank God for Chiropractic!

Lonnie — Santa Fe, NM

ॐ

I started chiropractic care in November of 1992. I was having constant lower back pain. I was unable to stand for more than two minutes. I selected a chiropractor who was highly recommended. I knew a good chiropractor could do me no harm and possibly save me from back surgery.

Chiropractic improved many of my physical conditions, including some I did not relate to back problems. They include increased circulation in my hands (they used to go numb for no reason), a restored regular heartbeat (no more palpations), easier breathing, bladder control improvement, a clear mind, improved sleeping, and of course, my back pain has improved to the point where I can walk and stand for longer periods of time without pain.

For all of the above reasons, I believe in chiropractic. I also feel my chiropractor made it possible for me to live not only a more normal life, but also a much improved quality over the last six months.

Carrie — Austin, TX

I'm afraid my story is not that of a miraculous cure. I first visited my chiropractor some six years ago when I was experiencing a muscle spasm in my back. Although heat, rest and muscle relaxants handled the immediate symptoms well enough, thanks to my sister's visits to her chiropractor in Montana, I realized that there might be something more involved. So I made a chiropractic appointment myself.

As soon as my chiropractor explained chiropractic to me, I became a believer. The physical relationship between subluxations and the sending of nerve impulses to the rest of the body is so obvious that I am truly amazed when everyone doesn't immediately jump on the chiropractic bandwagon.

My two daughters, fifteen and twelve, have also been getting adjusted for the last six years. As I mentioned, there have been no miracles. However, I do know that all three of us are healthy and recover rapidly when some small illness does strike. I enjoy the security of knowing when one of us falls over backward on a chair or lands resoundingly on her backside while roller skating, that our chiropractor will handle the resultant subluxations. Thirty years down the road, none of us will have to hang on a door to ease the pain of today's untreated vertebral problems.

Gene – Vancouver, WA

The most obvious benefit of chiropractic is of course the physical relief and strengthening that takes place. I find my lifestyle to be very physical. As a registered nurse, with my running everyday, I find there is a lot of pulling, pushing, and lifting. I feel this strain particularly in my neck, shoulder, and back. In the past, I would have taken two Tylenol, used heat, or some other medical remedy. Now I find relief is obtained because of my weekly adjustments.

A less obvious benefit is the decrease of tension I experience because of my weekly adjustments. As a priest, nurse, and counselor, I am exposed to conflict, stress, and anxiety on a regular basis. This exposure tends to make me feel some of these very same stressors.

Thanks to chiropractic, the physical benefits help restore a sense of inner harmony in conjunction with physical harmony. As a consequence of this I know that I function better because of chiropractic and I would highly recommend it to everyone.

Fr. Nathaniel – Los Angeles, CA

I was referred to a chiropractor by a friend who highly recommended I see him because of the fantastic results she was experiencing. I have had continuous pain in the right shoulder area for some time, and it was affecting my job, my fun time and my life!

The medical profession was not giving me resources to help me with my problem. I had medication for pain control but it made me sick to my stomach every time I took it. Chiropractic has taken away my pain. More importantly, I have been introduced to an entirely new philosophy of taking care of my body and maintaining good health. I am very sure this "way of good health" will work for me over the coming years!

Dana – Boise, ID

એ

I am a registered nurse and I worked in the hospital setting for several years. I was very discouraged, to say the least. It just didn't seem I was able to really help many people in that setting. All too often I couldn't believe what doctors were putting their patients through. I would always joke I would be the worlds worst patient because I wouldn't let a doctor do anything I wasn't positive I needed.

I wanted to help people prevent illness, not try to nurse them back to health using inadequate methods or comfort them to their death. Later, I worked at a clinic for non-life threatening emergencies and routine office visits. Several things amazed me and stunned me during that time.

The first was the number of people who came to the doctor for a cold or a flu, and who were given antibiotics for these viruses. Doctors and nurses know antibiotics don't help these conditions because they are used to fight bacteria, not viruses. Yet, they are still prescribed for these conditions. The second was the number of unnecessary X-rays and treatments that were done right before my eyes.

As a chiropractic patient for over 5 years, I know chiropractic works because it helped me with headaches and back pain. More importantly, it helped me with my overall health. It has also helped my family members in similar ways. I firmly believe that through regular chiropractic adjustments, my family and I will live longer, healthier lives and be better able to deal with the stresses that are so common to our daily routine.

Joan, RN/CA – Bethlehem, PA

When I became acquainted with chiropractic two years ago, I was at a point in my life when I wanted to assume responsibility for my body and health care. I had recently undergone surgery to remove my thyroid gland which had been disfunctional for six years. It was treated medically with drugs prior to the thyroidectomy in order to control symptoms of the disease. The drugs worked in terms of controlling symptoms. They effectively decreased the supply of thyroxin which was over stimulating my body functions.

However, this miracle of modern technology also had the ability to penetrate my placental wall, resulting in two pregnancies terminated in spontaneous abortions. Neither fetus could survive the effects of the drug responsible for maintaining a hormonal balance in my own body. I felt as though I was winning the battle, but losing the war.

I finally opted for surgery after which, I learned to my dismay, I was once again dependent on a drug. This drug was to replace the function of my thyroid gland by replenishing the absent hormone.

It was at this time I was first introduced to chiropractic. I felt healthy and knew I never wanted to "go under the knife" again. After being adjusted weekly for a year in order to maintain my body at an optimum level of function, I discovered I could decrease my medication with no ill effects. I finally discontinued the use of drugs completely after having the designated blood tests taken.

My medical doctor was amazed my thyroid gland has regenerated and was producing thyroxine at a normal rate.

I am now a healthy woman, free of the use of drugs and the fear chemical drugs could again interfere with the normal growth of a baby should I choose to become pregnant. Chiropractic care has given me a sense of permanent well-being and a brand new attitude toward life and health.

I am convinced regular adjustments along with sensible eating and a conscientious lifestyle, will maintain a healthy state of being.

Janet — Columbus, OH

My husband, Scott, suffered a serious back injury, and after seeking help from numerous medical professionals without relief, we finally ended up in a chiropractor's office.

We were struck immediately by the friendliness and the supportive, positive attitude of the staff. It was a breath of fresh air to receive the intelligent and sensitive answers to our questions after receiving mostly terse and minimal explanations from other medical doctors.

Best of all, we were impressed by the non-intervention, patient empowering philosophy espoused enthusiastically by our chiropractor, which coincides well with our own attitudes about health and wellness. Through the years we've gained an awareness of how crucial it is we take primary responsibility for our own well-being through a good diet and frequent exercise. Therefore, we mistrust the tenets of western medicine that the doctors will "cure" us. Baloney! We all must take care of ourselves.

After a couple of months of adjustments, Scott's pain subsided to the point he could return to his job as a carpenter. He had a stubborn problem, but our chiropractor remained a vital, positive, hopeful supporter during those weeks when the pain seemed omnipresent. We believe chiropractic care was central to Scott's recovery. Equally vital were the morning routine of back exercises and conscious relaxation throughout the day.

As for myself, both out of empathy and out of curiosity, I began chiropractic care. I didn't have any acute pain or condition, just aches and soreness at various points down my back. My experience, therefore, has been very different from Scott's. I have had no dramatic changes or recovery, just a slow, steady feeling over the months that I am stronger and healthier than ever. I do yoga and I have felt a definite improvement in my flexibility and endurance. The odd little "kinks" in my back when I would try certain postures are gone. In swimming, I seem to have all this new-found upper body strength and breathing capacity — I never swam so vigorously in my life!

Katie — Newark, NJ

Within 60 days of beginning chiropractic care strictly for wellness care purposes, 3 amazing problems disappeared. I recovered the hearing in my deaf ear. This is something several surgeons said would never happen. I regained the long lost ability to breathe through my nose at night. Lastly, but far from the least, I found the energy I thought was gone forever.

I recommend chiropractic wellness care to everyone I meet. The changes that can occur in your life are indefinite. Seeing a chiropractor was the wisest choice I ever made for my total health.

Dan – Salt Lake City, UT

≈

Before I began chiropractic care, there were numerous problems I was experiencing. For the past 11 years, I have been diagnosed with an autoimmune illness called Vasculitis. With this illness, I would continuously have a low-grade fever, a (itchy) rash and outbreak on my legs and to top it off, sinus problems and infections. I had begun to take medication for my sinuses and for the first time in September, 1996, I took Predisone for the Vasculitis. The Predisone did not take care of the elevated sedimentary rate or elevated liver function readings.

I started chiropractic care in late September at which time I felt conventional medicine was no longer a choice for me. This has been my best fall/winter season (the usual time of my maladies). I have not had a fever, I no longer take any prescription medicines, I am not experiencing any trouble with my legs (rash/outbreak), and next to no problems with my sinuses. One thing unrelated to the Vasculitis is that I have less to no problem with excessive stomach acid. This was an everyday occurrence in the past.

Thank you for delivering such a high quality product as chiropractic care.

Santo – Santa Clara, CA

A month and a half ago I was told I might need surgery to correct a bladder control problem. I was told by a friend who had the surgery that it was harder to recover from and more painful than her C-section. I've had the bladder problem for several years and it had become increasingly worse. Small amounts of urine would "leak" if I coughed, sneezed, laughed hard or squatted down.

Although I had forgot to mention this to my chiropractor, after the first few adjustments, the problem was correcting itself. This has made a drastic improvement in my life and I thank chiropractic for increasing my quality of life.

Joan   —   Martha's Vineyard, MA

ॐ

Before I made my first visit to a chiropractor I never knew the value of chiropractic care or how it would change my life. Since I have been under chiropractic care, I have noticed significant improvements in my health. Even though, I was informed it might take awhile to see the results, I noticed them within the first week of care.

I always internalized any stress in my life and as a result the muscles in my neck and shoulders were always tense. One of the most surprising things I noticed right away was I could sit or stand straight, shoulders back and chin up without any discomfort. In the past, I was very uncomfortable and my shoulders would always roll forward. Another surprise that came to me was my sense of smell became much more sensitive. I used to never be able to smell things unless they were directly in front of me.

The most important change that has happened and is still in progress is the hormonal balance returning to my reproductive system. I was diagnosed with endometriosis and advised I should take birth control pills to control my periods and eventually have an operation to clean out my system. Under chiropractic care, my periods are returning to normal and I have stopped taking birth control pills.

I still have a way to go before everything is back to normal but I feel great and for the first time in a very long time I have regained my positive outlook on life! I owe chiropractic a world of thanks, not just for the care but for the personalized care, support and positive energy it has provided me.

Lisa   —   Dallas, TX

I just wanted to briefly explain a phenomenon that occurred under chiropractic care. My husband and I had been trying to get pregnant for years with no results. After being under chiropractic care for just one month, it happened. I still can't believe it. I have heard chiropractic care has been beneficial in helping women with pregnancy problems, but I never thought it would help me.

Thank you so much. I will continue with a wellness care program under chiropractic care forever. God Bless!

Ginger – Atlanta, GA

Since I began chiropractic care, my stress level has been great and I can deal with situations in my life much easier than when I was constantly subluxated. I wake up in the morning with a lot more energy and peace of mind, not to mention a clearer mind.

I was dealing with Muscular Dystrophy and my spells have decreased, my vision has improved, the loss of balance I commonly experienced has drastically been reduced, and when I do feel a spell coming on I can mentally deal with it better than ever before.

Basically, I have a lot more energy and feel really great. I definitely feel I have a lot more to live for. Lastly, my eating habits have improved which makes life even more tolerable. Thanks!

Janet – Minneapolis, MN

Our family became acquainted with chiropractic care through our son, who was diagnosed as asthmatic at 2 and one-half years of age. He also has a central nervous system disorder that causes numerous symptoms including bouts of hyperactivity.

Within two adjustments, his asthma was gone and has not returned. Within six months of receiving chiropractic care, his hyperactivity was greatly diminished.

Our whole family now goes for regular adjustments under a chiropractic wellness care program. Our daughter had her first adjustment at 1 month old. Chiropractic has changed our lives by first changing our health...then our outlook on life.

Antonio & Andrea – NYC, NY

Prior to seeing a chiropractor, some of the bodily problems I had were:
   • Severe asthma causing me to always be on medication and inhalers
   • Pain up and down my entire spine
   • Cracking my neck and back was a habit because I was always in pain and cracking would help relieve some of the pain
   • Could not comfortably sit up straight with my shoulders back to promote good posture
   • Had to crack/pop my elbow up to 10 times a day to keep it from locking up
   • Walked with a slight limp due to one leg being shorter than the other
   • Woke up often during the night and could not sleep more than 5 or 6 hours, leaving me very tired, sluggish and not wanting to do anything

After I got tired of taking so many different medications to treat all of these symptoms, I decided to try something different. I have been seeing a chiropractor for two weeks and these are some of the changes I have noticed:
   • It is much easier for me to breathe, medication-free
   • My spine is pain-free except when I sit too long
   • I no longer need to crack my neck or back because of the adjustments to the spine, the pain is just about gone
   • I automatically sit up straight with my shoulders back
   • I only crack/pop my elbow 1 or 2 times a day out of habit
   • The limp is no longer noticeable because my legs are becoming more even
   • I no longer wake-up during the night and can sleep for 8 or 9 hours, leaving me feeling rested and ready for the day ahead of me
   Thanks for the great chiropractic care!

Deana – Vancouver, WA

I heard about chiropractic care from quite a few people at my church, including my pastor, Reverend Claude McNeely. Seeing the results so quickly makes me wish I did this as soon as I heard about chiropractic. I had been on a lot of medication for aches and pains in my body, as well as powerful medication for my asthma, which I have had for as long as I can remember.

After coming in for regular adjustments for about two months now, I can breath much better. I have been an asthmatic for as long as I can remember, so I am very happy about this improvement in my life. I feel better overall.

Before the chiropractic adjustments, I was taking drugs every day and now I do not need to any longer. No more Accolate for my asthma, or Tylenol for my head and back pains. I used to be sleepy, as well, before my regular chiropractic adjustments. I can now sleep better and when I am awake, I now have more energy than ever. I can also walk better and I feel lighter on my feet. I feel 20 years younger.

Seeing is believing and since I see the effects chiropractic adjustments have had on my overall wellness and fitness, it must be able to work on anyone.

Leo — Nashville, TN

è&

I was referred to a chiropractor by a friend of mine who was a chiropractic patient at the time. They had experienced positive results due to the specific adjustments, so I thought I would give it a whirl.

I was unable to put my own socks on or cleanse myself after a bowel movement. Once I started a chiropractic care program, I was able to perform these simple tasks so many take for granted.

Because of chiropractic, I am healthier, happier, and more knowledgeable. I now have a desire to help others to seek help for their spines.

Chiropractic took my pain away, made me feel good on a normal basis, and I now have the know-how to understand adjustments will help my body overcome troubles it experiences. Thank you for providing me with such exceptional care!

Timothy — Dayton, OH

When our daughter Sharon was a few months old, I went back to work and I had to get a babysitter. After several weeks of watching her, my first babysitter had to stop taking care of Sharon. Her problem was too much for the sitter to handle. Ever since Sharon was born she had bowel movement problems. Every time she had a bowel movement, we knew about it right away. She would cry and scream in pain. Immediately, her face would turn red and she would kick her feet until she was finished.

We naturally assumed something medically was wrong with her. The first doctor we took her to prescribed lime water and chamomile tea, but that did not work. The second doctor prescribed Xylocaine; that also failed. Finally, after a period of time passed, we couldn't think of anything else so we decided to try Children's Hospital to see if there was something they could do. We talked to a Lower GI Specialist. The doctor did a lower GI, a Barium Enema, and took X-rays to see if her colon was O.K. The X-rays turned out negative and everything was said to be working properly. The doctor said lots of kids do not like to go the bathroom and she would grow out of it.

One day my babysitter told me friends of hers mentioned chiropractic care might help. The chiropractor felt chiropractic could help the body overcome this problem Sharon was having. We didn't take her until about a month later. We felt if a medical doctor couldn't help her, what could a chiropractor do?

She was 13 months old when we brought Sharon to see the chiropractor for the first time. He informed us that the problem was in her lower back. It was very tight. A normal child would have been relaxed in that area.

For two months, we have had Sharon under chiropractic care. She would go twice a week to get her adjustments. Now, Sharon sees him once a week and in the near future, her visits will be cut down even more. Sharon is now 15 months old and going to the bathroom without pain.

It is so wonderful to see our baby's body functioning properly on its own from the chiropractic care she has received.

Mike & Theresa — Davenport, IA

I have experienced menstrual cramps and lower back pain for some time now. They have always put a serious hamper on my life. I knew it was not an incredibly unusual occurrence, but the pain I experienced was excruciating. I would take Tylenol for the pain. Finally, I got sick of taking the pain and I stopped by the building I had driven past so many times before.

That building was my new chiropractor's building. I have now been under care for just a few months and I no longer have such intense menstrual cramps. In fact, I barely get cramps at all. I just listen to my friends complain about theirs now.

My lower back rarely aches anymore. As a student, my lower back is under extreme stress (so many books to tote around) and I am extremely thankful to no longer have the pain.

I rarely believe anything unless I have seen it myself. I have felt what chiropractic and my chiropractor have done for me and that is proof enough for me. Chiropractic Works!

Sue – Chicago, IL

❧

In the past two months, since I have been under chiropractic care, there have been dramatic changes in my health, mind and marriage, which I must share.

At age 34, I had over ten years of suffering with hemorrhoids, chronic bladder infections and nauseous headaches. My neck and back were in constant discomfort and my general outlook on life was...well, let's not even discuss my general outlook on life. The specialists could find nothing wrong with me. I was diagnosed as having "irritable bowel syndrome" and "urethral syndrome." In 1989, I underwent two hemorrhoidectomies and was on continual medication since my marriage, as sex was determined to be a hazard to my bladder. This may also explain my poor outlook on life!

After only two weeks of chiropractic care, the bladder problems virtually disappeared and I am no longer taking regular medication. How happy I am to have found you! I cannot believe the difference feeling good makes in your life. I enjoy walking, sewing and good posture without pain. Thank you for being a caring professional!

Doreen – San Francisco, CA

I have had bronchial asthma for 18 years. I fell down steps at age 5 and broke my arm. Now I realize I didn't develop asthma until age 6. I came for chiropractic care a few times with backaches and then stopped care. After a few falls off a horse while horseback riding and a car accident, I started developing very sharp pains in my upper back, numbness in my arms and fingers, and chest pains.

My health started deteriorating. I developed kidney problems, my asthma started getting worse and I developed a lot of new allergies. After numerous trips to the medical doctor and being put on a number of medications that made me nauseated and constantly tired, I remembered being told by a chiropractor that asthma and allergies respond very well to chiropractic adjustments.

I knew this was my last hope, so I sat down and went through my background history and started chiropractic care immediately. At first it was rough because I had some dizziness, nausea and pain. However, after my chiropractor explained that my body had been ill for so long and it was going through a lot of change, I understood what was happening. My chiropractor explained if I didn't keep up my regular adjustments I would be right back where I started from.

I did not want that to happen again, so I kept up with all of my appointments and have not had a kidney problem since. My asthma still acts up a little bit, and just having relief from it is a blessing. Relief from illness without the side effects from medication is an even bigger blessing.

Eve - Morrisville, PA

> ## *"Get knowledge of the spine, for this is the requisite for many diseases."*
>
> — Hippocrates

I f I believed in miracles, I would state that my chiropractor has per-formed one. However, I realize what you have done for me is the result of years of serious study and experience in the field of chiro-practic, plus constant vigilance in keeping up-dated with new develop-ments in a field that furnishes, for me at least, an application of logic and common sense.

I have found in you, more than a doctor, however. I have come to accept you as a great friend, a wise philosopher, and a most caring and understanding person. Let me explain what I refer to as a "miracle."

At the rather ripe age of 85 years, I have been experiencing several of the more or less common ailments that come to many of us...arthri-tis, urinary infection, and lower circulatory deficiency. The medical profession has done little for any of these diseases except treat, in the case of the urinary problem, the symptom through the repeated use of anti-biotics and recommending surgery.

Recently, the leg problem has become a threat to my continued lifestyle. The medical experts have tested and re-tested and come up with the conclusion that the veins are calcified; a condition for which they offer no remedy except possibly eventually amputation of the legs.

I relayed this information to my chiropractor and he went to work on adjustments that would improve the condition. The bottom line is the urinary infection has never recurred, the arthritis is checked, and most remarkable of all, the condition of my legs has significantly start-ed to improve to the point I no longer feel doomed to lose the degree of quality of life that previously confronted me. What a relief!

Gil – Spokane, WA

I started bringing my four year old daughter to a chiropractor when a friend suggested it may help with her bladder and kidney infection. In May of 1997, Mackenzie had her first appointment. After meeting the chiropractor, I became hopeful he may also be able to help her with a sleep disorder, headaches and some eczema Mackenzie had also been suffering from.

Right from the beginning, Mackenzie enjoyed her visits with the chiropractor. She told me she felt better after her adjustments. After a few weeks we began to notice Mackenzie was able to finally sleep through the night (something she has never done before). Mackenzie also stopped complaining about headaches and she hasn't developed any patches of eczema and our original complaint of very frequent urination and lack of bladder control has improved greatly. I am confident with continued care, Mackenzie will continue to improve.

Since we started chiropractic care, I've also noticed Mackenzie's overall outlook on life has improved greatly. She is much happier and generally a more relaxed child. As she continues to improve and she continues to look forward to her adjustments, I look forward to seeing the many positive changes in my daughter both physically and emotionally.

Mari Jo & Mackenzie   —   Port Elgin, Ontario, Canada

Aside from the obvious back problem (and neck) when I first made the acquaintance with my chiropractor, there was a very definite problem with my nervous system. I had discussed it with any and every doctor I ever made contact with. I read any article I came across that I thought may give me a clue. I spoke to nurses, interns and nutritionists. No one had any answers for me. In my mind, I was convinced whatever it was that was wrong, was someday going to rear its ugly head and render me disabled and by that time be beyond treatment. I felt it would be a dystrophy of some sort.

To explain what I felt is difficult. It seemed to me to be a sort of spin off from cramps in my legs. I was a victim of very severe cramps for years. They started to be severe in the early seventies. Cramps were a problem for me ever since I was young, but about then they were starting to keep me up walking the floor at night. Shin splints were common to me and at times, I would jump into the tub just to run very warm water over my legs. Hoping for relief, I ate bananas, citrus, etc. I put electric blankets on my legs, I wore sweatpants and sometimes two pairs of socks to bed.

By the time I sought chiropractic care in December of 1988, there was just nothing else to do. Still, as soon as I relaxed they were there. At that time I was getting cramps anywhere in my body, not only in my legs. If I unscrewed a lid that was tight or held the wheel of the car too long in one position, my hand would cramp (just like a charlie horse). If I reached for something, my legs, toes, stomach, side and arm would cramp. It was incredible and quite bizarre. Believe it or not - even my tongue would cramp in my throat.

It is hard to associate time so far as years but I would say about 1980 I started to have sensations that seemed to me to have a direct connection to the cramps. When I sat down or was off my feet for any reason there was "something" going on in my muscles. It could be anywhere but mostly in my legs and buttocks. To put it very simply it felt like I had dozens of little worms moving around. It didn't hurt at all. It was like an electric current running through me. Thank God I never felt it in my head. I would have really gone crazy! It seemed to strike anywhere but never my head.

I knew this was going to take me some time to explain. I hope I have not bored you with the details, but maybe you can understand why I felt it could only get worse and I would eventually be incapacitated.

In 1987, my neck and back were so bad, I couldn't walk straight, especially when I first got out of bed. I had tennis elbow in both arms.

I was missing so much work because of vanity. If I couldn't walk upright, I didn't want to be seen. At 50, I felt as though I was practicing to be 80.

My son kept telling me to see a Chiropractor. "No," I didn't want someone "cracking my bones." Finally, after many Doctor bills I gave up. I felt I had to accept the inevitable. I was not going to be one of those people who aged gracefully. I was going to be 50 and look 80! I didn't know it then but I wasn't desperate enough yet.

Come November of 1988, I couldn't bear the thought of facing a new year feeling as I did without giving it one more try. I made an appointment with a chiropractor.

Today I walk straight and in all honesty, the sensations I had that were driving me crazy are gone! I have a couple cramps from time to time but they never get me out of bed anymore. It isn't a miracle. It is chiropractic care. It isn't magic, and it can't be accomplished in 5, 15 or X amount of adjustments. It's ongoing care that is very necessary for me.

I don't know that any other doctor could have given me this state of mind. You are so unique! You believe in yourself, your ability and your art. I'm sure you don't look at what you do as "art," but you see, with you it is. Your skill, your personality, your love of people, your desire to help, is all tied together in what you do, and that my dear, dear friend is art to me.

Rudy - Trenton, NJ

> *"... a kind of super intelligence exists in each of us, infinitely smarter and possessed of technical know-how far beyond our present understanding."*
>
> — Lewis Thomas, M.D.

I'm 52 years old and have had a long history of health problems (insomnia, high blood pressure, irregular bowels, sinusitis, renoids syndrome, noise sensitivity, bizarre dreams, weak hips and knees plus what my grandmother referred to as "widows hump"). These problems stemmed from several childhood accidents and illnesses.

Back in the 1970's, I went to a chiropractor who told me he couldn't help me because of a back injury I'd had when I was younger. So I started going to one doctor after another. By the time I finally returned to receive chiropractic care, I was in extreme pain and my medical doctors were saying I'd need hip and knee surgeries soon. I was also popping Ibuprofen like candy.

My chiropractor has an office next to my work and a lot of his patients would come in and tell me how he'd helped them and how great they felt. Finally, in May of 1992, I went in and got set up for chiropractic care.

Within just a few weeks, I could see and feel I'd come a long, long way on the road to quality living. In fact, when I saw my X-rays, I couldn't find any evidence why I would need surgery. It was really enlightening.

At any rate, constant pain was becoming a thing of the past and I was sleeping 8-10 hours a night, plus, I was walking taller and bouncier than I ever had in my life. Even now, my family can't believe the changes in me. I really do feel great and my weekly "tune-ups" (adjustments) make me feel like I'm on Cloud Nine.

Many of my family members are now under chiropractic care and have experienced notable changes in their lives. Many of my friends and acquaintances are also using my chiropractor with great results. I'll say it again and again how great I feel and how much I have been helped -in all areas-by my chiropractor. I just wish I would have got a second opinion years ago.

It's been so long since I've taken an Ibuprofen that I can't remember when I stopped. Thank You So Much!

Anne — Bethesda, MD

I would like to tell you about my son, Kevin. He is 7 1/2 years old and has been coming to a chiropractor for about six weeks. When Kevin was 3 years old, he was diagnosed as having Attention Deficit Hyperactivity Disorder (ADHD). After trying diet changes, allergy testing, and behavioral modification techniques, we reluctantly agreed to put Kevin on Ritalin. The medication did its job as far as slowing him down a little bit, but he suffered from many side effects.

In two years he grew only two inches and did not gain any weight at all. He cried easily, had trouble sleeping, no appetite and would zone out quite often. Finally, at age 6 we made the decision to stop giving him Ritalin. He grew six inches in less than one year and gained nearly 15 pounds. His sleeping and eating patterns were still erratic and his school work was horrible. He had a teacher with a lot of energy and patience which helped him somewhat but he still could not sit still, his writing was illegible, and math made no sense to him. He was still struggling.

That is where Kevin was at before we brought him in for chiropractic care. He was seen twice a week for six weeks. This last week when I went to his parent/teacher conference, the first thing his teacher asked me was, "had we put Kevin back on Ritalin." I said, "No," and she pulled out samples of Kevin's work and showed me the sudden improvement in what he was able to do. For the first time, his handwriting is on the lines, it is much easier to read and much more age-appropriate. Although he still tends to move around more than the average child, he is able to concentrate, answer questions correctly and is reading better than most of his class. Chiropractic works!

Sometimes the results are sudden and dramatic like Kevin's experience, but more often the changes are slow and steady over time. The important thing is chiropractic allows the body to function at its best without interference from spinal misalignments. Drugs do not heal the body, they hinder the body from healing itself. Being adjusted regularly has literally changed my son's life. Thank You!

Barbara — Solano Beach, CA

As I was growing up, it seemed like everyday I had something wrong with me. We'd be at the doctor's office one day for an ear infection, get an antibiotic to treat the symptoms and the day after I would finish the medication, I would be back in the doctor's office with another ear infection. It was like an on-going cycle that just wouldn't stop.

A few years later, at about the age of 5, I found out I had asthma which was probably triggering the ear infections. My allergies got so bad, I had to get allergy shots, take an inhaler, use a peakflow, and nose spray and live on allergy medicine.

We had heard of chiropractic care, and how effective it was, so we decided to give it a try.

We made an appointment with a chiropractor in November 1995. After my first few adjustments I felt much better. I actually knew what normal felt like.

Eventually, I got off the allergy shots, the inhaler, peakflow, nose sprays and the allergy medicines too.

Now at the age of 12, during the first actual full year of going to the chiropractor, I received PERFECT ATTENDANCE for my sixth grade year. I feel I owe this award to my chiropractor, who kept me healthy throughout the year through chiropractic adjustments.

There will never be a doubt in my mind that chiropractic care is the reason my family and I are so healthy.

Billie – Puyallup, WA

ࢢ

Our son Thomas was born on September 22, 1989. His rate of development was slow, but still within normal parameters. He smiled, made the usual baby noises and was a happy, healthy child. We became concerned when his verbal skills had not emerged by the age of two. By that time, he had even stopped saying mama and dada. Our pediatrician suggested Tom suffered from global development delays. Shortly after this diagnosis, we moved to Connecticut and subsequently enrolled Tom in an early intervention program at age 3. Following a short period in this program, Tom was finally diagnosed with autism (by Yale) in March 1995.

Prior to age 3, Tommy had not exhibited any autistic symptoms of which we were aware. However, from age 3 on, several symptoms started appearing and grew markedly worse in spite of early intervention. These symptoms include self-stimulation (twiddling a sock between his fingers), echolalia PICA, lack of socialization skills, aggression, sleep disturbances, mild self abuse, frequent temper tantrums, and lack of interest in toys. In September 1995, we decided to place Tommy in a special education inclusion program at a neighboring elementary school. Under the guidance of a wonderful special education teacher, Tommy showed improvement in his social skills, verbal skills and cognitive development. However, his aggression, PICA and temper tantrums continued to worsen.

His aggressiveness had increased to such an extent that it was decided to enlist the help of a behavioral psychologist. An effective behavior modification program was finally instituted in July, 1996. His decreased aggression facilitated more positive interaction, especially between Tommy and his 10 year old sister. However, his other autistic symptoms were still very prevalent.

We have read many books on autism in an attempt to help our son as much as possible. In all the information we have found, there was not one mention that chiropractic could be a tool in caring for autistic children. When a friend told me of the successes her chiropractor had with children with special needs, we decided it was worth trying. The fact that chiropractic is non-invasive and drug-free made it especially attractive.

We made an appointment with this chiropractor in November, 1996. The day after his first adjustment was the best day Tommy has ever had! He played with toys all day and was very calm and his interactive speech increased dramatically. He played with his sister! The change in him has been truly remarkable. Although he still has his ups and downs, his downs have been much less severe.

Overall, the improvement in his cognitive and social development has been dramatic. He is now learning to read! His participation in his general education class has gone from 70% in October 1996 to 86% in February 1997. His classmates interact with him to a much greater extent. He also eats a wider variety of foods; and sleep disturbances have been reduced.

There is no doubt in our minds chiropractic has been instrumental in reducing Tommy's autistic symptoms.

The Bauer Family – Hartford, CT

This letter was written by a victim of a car accident/chiropractic patient to another victim of a car accident.

My name is Brett Armstead. I am 31 years old and I was told about your situation with your accident and I'm here to tell you how important chiropractic care is and how much it will help you.

I have been involved in two car accidents recently, neither of them my fault. In the first accident, I was stopped at a traffic light and I was rear ended by a young woman. I severely injured my neck and lower back. I went through every medical doctor possible; orthopedic surgeons, family physicians, therapists, etc. and none of them helped me. They put me on pain medications and that helps to take away some of the pain temporarily. My spine was totally out of whack! This was creating all of the problems.

I was finally in enough pain to go to the chiropractor. After one visit, I noticed improvement in my neck and lower back. After about 12 visits, I actually felt like myself again, with practically no pain! I continued on a maintenance program and I felt great!

Unfortunately, on 07/04/94, I was involved in another car accident. This time I was hit head on by a drunk driver. I now have two bulging discs in my back, and neck problems from the accident.

Since the accident, I have been under chiropractic care and without it, I know I would not be out of bed yet. I am now back to lifting weights four times a week and I am able to get back to all of my regular activities.

I guess what I am trying to get through to you, is that if you have been involved in a serious car accident, you may have underlying problems you may not have symptoms from yet. You may not feel the effects of these problems until you are 31 like myself. Don't wait! Take care of your body now. Chiropractic care has been the best choice I have ever made!

Brett   —   St. Louis, MO

Case Studies — Part 1

The following four testimonials were recorded and written by the passionate chiropractic patient, David Hanger, in Tauranga, New Zealand. These case studies originated from the Chiropractic in New Zealand Report.

"My Chiropractic Child"

In all respects, the birth of Glennis and Terry Luke's fifth child, Derek, conformed with all that the medical profession of the day would term a "normal induced birth."

Convinced over the objections of the mother, of over-term status, doctors instructed that on the morning of October 31, 1973, the birth be induced.

Fourteen hours later, after just two hours of labor, the doctor-assisted birth came to a "satisfactory" conclusion.

Having been through it all four times before, Glennis and Terry, ecstatically happy about the addition to their close family unit, accepted the medical procedures without undue concern.

Terry was not there to witness the pulling and twisting, the virtual assault on the emerging baby's neck and upper spine, as the Resident, using Derek's head as a handle, "assisted" nature's work and hastened the arrival in the then traditional manner.

The tiny, still forming vertebrae protecting the spinal cord, conduit for the vital nervous system, was in the process placed under great - and probably damaging - strain.

Within hours it was discovered the new born was afflicted with jaundice.

The discovery caused no alarm to doctors or the parents. Three of Luke's other children had also been touched by jaundice.

In each case, the malady had quickly disappeared.

Even when, after three days without noticeable improvement, the hospital authorities decided to place Derek under intensive care, no great concern was felt.

The modern city hospital, well-equipped and serving a population of 100,000 or more, handled many such cases with complete confidence and almost certain success.

Glennis signed over the care of her baby to the hospital knowing he would come under the supervision of eminently qualified medical people.

Routinely, Derek was stripped and placed in a cot beneath the light-healing fluorescent tubes hanging about a meter above his jaundiced body.

Farmer Terry and the rest of the family carried on their lives much the same as usual. In the hospital maternity wing, Glennis regained her strength and contentedly awaited for the time her newborn would be returned to her side.

It did not happen.

Derek, suffering three times a day the knife prick in his heel to obtain blood samples, failed to respond to the light treatment, his bilirubin count hovering around the dangerous 15 level.

Any rise above that level, Glennis was told, would require an immediate blood transfusion. The count in fact rose to 20, but no blood transfusion was attempted.

As the days went by, Derek became more irritable, sleeping for only two hours at a time, then demanding to be fed.

Glennis, now ready to go home, fretted over the fact that on too many occasions she arrived to breast feed her baby only to discover nurses had already done it for her with expressed milk.

Then came the day when she was told part of Derek's problem arose through his incompatibility with her milk.

To Glennis, the news was devastating. She had breast fed all her previous children and she desperately wanted to give Derek an equal start in life.

But who was she to argue with the authority of the hospital's chief pediatrician? All she could do was plead her case — and suffer the stern rejection.

Derek, she was told, would go on to the bottle while Glennis went through the emotionally painful process of drying up her natural milk supply.

By the tenth day, both Glennis and Terry experienced a growing unease about the welfare of their baby son, their distress reaching out to infect the rest of the family happiness at the great event being replaced by anguish and worry.

Expressions of concern directed by the Lukes' with hospital personnel were brushed aside with what was in those days the usual professional disdain.

"You can't expect miracles to occur overnight you know. Everything possible is being done. You must learn patience. Let the healing process take its course," experts advised.

After 12 days, family discussions turned around the desirability of obtaining chiropractic aid.

Over the years, the Luke family had experienced great benefit from the services of Tauranga's veteran chiropractor, Dr. David McCarthy.

First they took their fears to their respected family doctor, consulted originally as a matter of course when the pregnancy first became evident.

He advised his patients that he no longer had control over Derek's progress, this having been taken away from him when the Lukes were required to sign responsibility for Derek's medical care over to the hospital.

However, he did concede he could see no harm coming from a chiropractic examination.

The Luke's family medical advisor was at that time one of the very few medical people in the country who were prepared to recognize the value of chiropractic care.

But he knew he must tread carefully, for under the strictures of the powerful New Zealand Medical Association prevailing at the time, he could face severe disciplinary action if he should dare to go so far as to recommend chiropractic involvement in this case.

On the thirteenth day of Derek's life - ten of them having been spent almost exclusively under the glare of fluorescent lights - Terry gained the attention of the hospital pediatrician and put to him the proposal of chiropractic care.

The pediatrician's reaction was entirely predictable. He totally rejected any chiropractic "interference."

He declared there was no sound reason to consider a second opinion outside the hospital, from any source whatsoever.

Derek, he claimed, was already receiving the best possible medical treatment available to anyone anywhere in the country.

Slow to anger but nevertheless formidable when roused, Terry responded to the frustration coursing through him and many harsh words were said on both sides.

That night, around the family dining room table, the decision was made — they would take their baby to their chiropractor, come what may.

The idea of Dr. McCarthy visiting the hospital in his professional capacity was not discussed. Both parties knew full well that such a happening, as desirable as it may be, was not possible under the rules of the medical association controlling the hospital staff's actions.

Instead, Dr. McCarthy wrote a letter to the pediatrician at the request of the Lukes, in which he said in part: "I do not ask that you endorse a chiropractic examination, nor give approval to take the baby to a chiropractor. I do however, ask that if it is the wish of these good folk to bring their baby to me and have him checked over, then I ask you do not make it difficult for them.

"If it transpires they do bring their baby to me for treatment I would be interested to know the changes, if any, in the subsequent blood tests."

Three years later, Dr. McCarthy's letter became part of the Commission of Inquiry records.

The last sentence of his letter obviously indicates Dr. McCarthy had in mind that Derek be taken back to the hospital immediately following chiropractic examination and care.

On the fourteenth day, Terry and Glennis arrived at the hospital determined to take Derek to Dr. McCarthy for examination.

The hospital staff was equally determined that no such heretical action would happen.

Among the ploys used was that of detailing the extreme danger Derek would be subjected to if he was removed from 24-hour-a-day monitoring.

The couple were brutally told if they removed Derek there was a good chance he would suffer brain damage.

In a just-in-case-chiropractic-works declaration, it was announced that that very day Derek had shown signs of improvement, so much so that the taking of blood samples had stopped, at least temporarily.

It was later revealed that so bruised and battered were Derek's heels, sit of the three-times a day blood letting, that it had been decided it would be wise to forego blood sampling for at least one day.

The Lukes were told by a now out-of-control medic that they were totally irresponsible and that a court injunction would be taken out against them requiring they give up guardianship of the child in favor of the hospital authorities.

Finally came the most stunning blow of all: "If you remove this baby from my care, then I don't want to see him back in this hospital for at least three months," raged the pediatrician in charge.

Glennis, with tears in her eyes and reeling from the impact of those terrible words, but carried forward by the love and support of her husband Terry, walked out of the hospital carrying in her arms their unhappy and sick child.

The heartache and anguish was evident to all who witnessed this sad scene.

As the small group left the hospital bound for Dr. McCarthy's clinic, the Lukes were handed a note in which it was recorded that the baby was being removed from the hospital against medical advice and possible brain damage could result.

This note was later also to become part of the Commission of Inquiry records.

As the trio traveled across town, the enormity of what they had done began to dawn on them, as realization came, so did the fear for their child's life.

In a country renowned throughout the world for its quality of professional hospital services, open to all its citizens at absolutely no cost to the patient, a place of healing where sufferers could depend on prompt and caring service at any hour of the day or night, this 14-day-old baby had, in their understanding, been barred from entry for a term of three months.

Why had their child been singled out to suffer such a harsh sentence?

Because they had dared to seek the second opinion of a health practitioner, fully licensed and registered under the law of the land, but who was outside the pale of services recognized by the all-powerful New Zealand Medical Association.

In Dr. McCarthy's clinic, the next act of this amazing drama began to unfold. Gently lying Derek face down on a couch, Dr. McCarthy drew his experienced and highly sensitive fingers along the baby's spine.

Using a sophisticated heat-sensitive instrument, he saw the flickering needle on the micro-calibrated dial confirm his manual discovery of a dysfunctioning vertabra — in chiropractic terms, a vertebral subluxation.

The dysfunction was in that area of the spine from which exited the nerves controlling the function of the liver, source of the malfunction causing jaundice. Perhaps a slight pressure on the nerves was resulting in a less than 100 percent filtration of the blood as it passed through the liver.

Perhaps the release of the pressure may possibly allow the infant body to correct its liver malfunction.

A carefully controlled, but dynamic palm thrust on the offended joint completed the care — without a flicker of protest from the tiny patient.

The examination and care had taken less than 20 minutes. The Lukes were free to take their baby away from the clinic, with another appointment set down for the Wednesday of the following week.

Within hours of taking their baby home, both Glennis and Terry noticed a dramatic improvement in his general wellbeing.

The tenseness had gone, the irritability reduced and a more natural, relaxed state had enveloped their son.

After feeding, Derek slept for four hours straight, the longest he had since birth. Over the weekend, there was more improvement.

By Tuesday, four days after the first adjustment by Dr. McCarthy, the skin had all but returned to normal.

Ten days after the first visit to the chiropractor's clinic, all signs of jaundice had disappeared.

Although only three adjustments had been performed in that time, Dr. McCarthy kept in daily contact with the Lukes to ensure no relapse had occurred.

On two or three occasions, he traveled out to the farm to see for himself how things were going. In keeping with his usual practice of maintenance after initial care, Dr. McCarthy continued to give the now healthy baby regular adjustments for about two months.

Glennis and Terry happily number themselves among those enlightened human beings who seldom find the need to visit their medical doctor.

They fully appreciate the value of maintaining a healthy body. One of the requirements to that end being a drug-free, uncluttered nervous system able to cope on its own with bodily dysfunctions.

Their chiropractor, Dr. David McCarthy proved to their certain satisfaction that his professional knowledge and expert care has greatly improved their lives. He kept those vital nerve passages clear for the entire family for many years, and his chiropractic sons carried on after he passed away.

The Lukes know chiropractic works. It works because they have made it a habit to straighten out the kinks before the kinks begin to destroy the nerve functions, thus affecting the organs they serve.

Glennis and Terry are blissfully unaware that the incidence of vertebral subluxation is now recognized by world scientific authorities as the most prolific epidemic of the 20th century, an epidemic likely to spill over into the 21st century unless the negative influence of medicine and drug companies is overcome.

They are unaware of this terrible plight on human development because they themselves, over many years of chiropractic care, have come to enjoy the benefits of a trouble-free spine. Their children have even more of a chance.

Their children's children, born without the hereditary bodily handicaps passed on by afflicted parents, will undoubtedly achieve even greater personal development as they progress in harmony with others similarly enhanced.

"Condemned to a Wheelchair"

When this story was first published as a Chiropractic under oath pamphlet, Patrick Sheehy, 38 years of age and the father of two fine children, was a happily married man, holding down a responsible job with a government department.

Seeing him then it was hard to accept that at 18 years of age he left the Oamaru Hospital in a wheel chair, deeply troubled by the farewell words of his medical advisers.

They said he would never walk again; that the ever present headaches and the wheel chair would be his constant companions for the rest of his life.

They said he should be moving north to the country's only hospital spinal care unit in Auckland, there to come under the charge of hospital staff specially trained to care for the permanently disabled.

Instead, he was going home because his widowed mother would have nothing to do with the proposed journey north.

Six months earlier, his life had hung in the balance as he went from one medical crisis to another, his body still rebelling against the violence of a traffic accident suffered at the age of 15.

At one point, the surgeon in charge of his case called in Paddy's mother and informed her that her son was slipping fast and could well die within 24 hours.

"A lot of people were praying for me at this time and I am sure their prayers helped me pull through that and many other crises," he told the writer during the researching of his incredible story.

As he will tell anyone willing to listen, it was the skill of an Oamaru Chiropractor which paved the way for his remarkable recovery.

The chiropractor's skill, coupled with his own religious convictions enabled the transformation of his battered body from that of a physical wreck, depending on a man-made contraption for mobility, to that of a normal family man living a full and meaningful life.

In Paddy's case, the "miracle" followed a vehicle accident in 1961. The car he was in collided with a power pole. Paddy, after first projecting part way through the front windscreen, rebounded back into the car and was immediately propelled through the side window, coming into violent contact with the power pole.

There followed a period of two-and-a-half years in the hospital.

During this time he underwent innumerable tests and a vast variety of treatments, all prescribed in the hope of overcoming the severe headaches and restoring the use of his lower limbs.

Among other things, the doctors performed a series of lumbar punctures, arteriograms, EEG tests and took a number of X-rays. For a short period he was transferred to the neurosurgical unit in Dunedin where, as he told the commissioners, "Presumably, a blood clot was removed from my brain."

He further testified that while the brain surgery relieved the pressure caused by the blood clot, his condition became further complicated by a total loss of balance, apparently as a result of the surgery.

"I discovered it was impossible to support my own body weight, even in a chair," he testified.

"I was examined by many specialists. None could provide an explanation for the headaches or the paralysis."

During hospitalization, his left foot became badly twisted and there was gross wasting of his leg muscles.

Having exhausted all avenues of treatment, the hospital authorities eventually decided there was nothing more they could do. It was either the Auckland Hospital's Spinal Care Unit or home, they said.

Although both Paddy and his mother decided to make the best of it in their Oamaru home, there were times when he doubted the wisdom of that decision.

"Conditions at our house were not geared to cope with a paraplegic," the witness told the commission.

"Trying to cope with a paraplegic without facilities or outside aid nearly broke my mother's back and her heart."

"My mother really was not strong enough to care for a crippled teenager," he said.

"She was living on a pension, as I was, so there was little chance to get out and about."

"Going to the toilet was a major project. It was outside. The wheel chair would not go through the back door, so it was necessary for me to drag myself outside every time I wanted to go to the toilet."

On the witness stand, Dr. Sim, a chiropractor, described how Paddy would drag himself into the waiting room, "Leaving a trail of dirty marks across the floor. Then he would hoist himself into a chair and sit there and wait his turn."

There was much about this case which surprised Dr. Sim.

"The most amazing thing he told me was that he could ride a horse. I thought he was a 'nut' to try that sort of thing, but he could do it."

Progress was slow and often painful for Paddy. But the persistence of the chiropractor and the positive responses of the patient were a powerful healing force.

A year after chiropractic care began, Paddy, at the suggestion of Dr. Sim, called on a medical doctor he knew and asked for a physical checkup.

The doctor, who had been aware of the earlier seemingly hopeless condition, conducted a lengthy medical examination.

Paddy testified that the medical doctor had been astounded at his own diagnosis. "He declared he couldn't find anything wrong with me," Paddy said.

While on the stand, Dr. Sim described in some detail the technical nature of the vertebral subluxations which had caused the paralysis.

He also described the care he adopted to correct the twisted foot.

He explained to the commissioners that much of the problem had been brought about by impaired but reversible nerve supply, a condition which an adjustment had been able to correct.

In the early stages of care, the Oamaru Hospital authorities learned of the chiropractic involvement.

They were not pleased.

When Paddy asked the hospital for walking equipment, it was refused.

When he improved still further and requested crutches, that request too was rejected.

On each occasion, others came to the rescue with the required equipment. Eventually, he was able to discard all aids for mobility.

His rapid recovery was aided to a degree by the fact that before the accident he had been a keen sportsman and had kept his body in good shape.

Just before the accident, he was confidently looking forward to a successful career as an amateur boxer.

It was natural that once he had regained his mobility, Paddy immediately reintroduced a regular training program.

He told the commissioners he had not suffered a day's illness since the completion of that initial period of chiropractic care.

He was able, he explained, to get secure employment in the Ministry of Agriculture as a meat inspector, a job which requires him to stay on his feet for up to 14 hours a day during the busy part of the season.

In October, 1984, Paddy reported to the author that he had that month participated, for the first time in his life, in a road race.

Held in Oamaru, the race was over a 10 kilometer course and more than 260 runners took part.

With obvious pride, Paddy declared he had come ahead of more than 200 runners to gain 56th place.

"Considering I couldn't even stand when the medical people gave up on me that's quite an achievement for chiropractic, wouldn't you say?" he said.

The writer would add: And it's also quite an achievement for faith, self-determination and sheer courage on the part of Paddy Sheehy.

"A Memory Restored"

Alison Money, while still at school, suffered severe mental incapacity following an accident in which her head came in violent contact with a concrete footpath.

The medical profession, apart from performing surgery to remove a blood clot, were unable to offer any solutions to Alison's loss of memory, depression, mood changes and generally very poor state of health.

Many years after the accident, Alison visited a chiropractor.

Alison's story was one of those presented, under oath, to the New Zealand Royal Commission of Inquiry into Chiropractic, and consequently became part of the report to the government which recommended chiropractic be treated as an equal health partner to the medical profession.

Her story follows.

Alison Money, about to celebrate her 12th birthday, was an above average student at the Taita (Wellington, New Zealand) Intermediate School. More often than not her examination results were among the top half dozen of around 30 students.

Alison was also glowingly fit and healthy. Like many an exuberant child she had a habit of moving about the school grounds on the run.

At the end of the school day on December 4, 1962, Alison headed for the bicycle stand in preparation for cycling home. As usual her pace could only be described as a headlong dash. And why not? All was well with the world. This happy, bright, vivacious young girl had every reason to be full of the joys of life.

Before her, two elder sisters had both done well at school. Her three-year-old sister was on the way to following the family tradition. The Moneys on that fateful day were a well adjusted, happy family going about their respective normal lives.

The young lad, about the same age as Alison, charging out of his classroom, also had every right to be full of the joys of life. He too was in a hurry as he began his journey home. Just outside the door the boy and the girl met. It was a disastrous meeting for Alison.

Caught off balance she began to fall. As she fell her body twisted around so she came to rest sprawled on her back on the ground, her head having come in violent contact with the concrete footpath. For those who noticed this event it was just another example of over-energetic children getting in each other's way.

The boy, unhurt, bounced to his feet and continued happily on his way, blissfully unconcerned and unaware of the catastrophic consequences which were to come from his violent, if fleeting contact with Alison Money.

Always an independent soul, Alison slowly and painfully picked herself up. Although in tears, badly shaken and suffering from a pounding headache, she doggedly stumbled over to her bicycle and rode home.

By the time she arrived there the shock of the accident had to a certain extent abated. Instead of telling her mother what had happened, she went straight upstairs and lay down on her bed.

Mrs. Thelma Money, going about her own affairs, called out a greeting to Alison as the child quietly made her way up the stairs. She did not notice anything was amiss. Had she stopped to think about it, she very likely would have realized as time went on that Alison was not as much in evidence as she usually was after she came home from school each day. During the evening meal, Alison was quieter than usual, and ate little. But it was not until around 10 p.m. that the horror began. Crying out in pain, Alison staggered down the stairs holding her head in her hands.

Her mother, of course, had no idea what was wrong, but she knew whatever it was it was serious. Mrs. Money immediately telephoned the family's medical doctor. As fate would have it their usual medical adviser was that date not on duty. However, his practice partner said he would come immediately.

By the time the medical man arrived, Alison had quieted down. But she was still obviously very sick. The doctor questioned Alison and learned of the accident at school.

He could find nothing obviously wrong, so prescribed aspirin and said the Money's own medical doctor would call in the morning. Mrs. Money gained the impression the doctor felt she had overstated the problem when first ringing through to the surgery.

That night is a night the Moneys will never forget. There was no sleep for any member of the family as Alison alternated between screaming from the pain in her head and vomiting as her whole body rebelled against the trauma taking place throughout her nervous system.

Next morning, when the doctor arrived as promised, Alison was in a semi-conscious state, obviously exhausted and seriously ill. Without preamble the doctor arranged for an immediate transfer to the local hospital.

Forty-eight hours later they operated to remove, they said, a blood clot in the brain.

A little over two months later they sent Alison home, the medical people advising Thelma Money it was unlikely Alison would ever return to a normal state.

Yes, they said, there was definitely something wrong with Alison's mental stability. She appeared, they said, to have undergone a dramatic and detrimental change of character as a result of the head injury.

They added that Alison was still emotionally unstable and would probably remain so. There was nothing more they could do. The family was told they must learn to live with the situation.

A few months later, Alison went back to school.

But this was not the Alison Money of the term before. No longer did she dash about the school grounds. Her teachers soon discovered Alison was no longer to be considered one of their brighter pupils. In fact, Alison very rapidly slid down in her grading to the bottom of the class. But no one did anything to help her overcome her handicap.

From intermediate school, in accordance with establishment procedures, she moved to Taita College, there to struggle through every day's schooling, scarcely able to remember a thing the teachers were telling her.

Eventually she reached the age of 15 when she could legally leave what to her had become the hated school regime.

Alison's mother was to testify 14 years later to the New Zealand Commission of Inquiry into Chiropractic that Alison had gained absolutely nothing from those last three years at school.

Then followed eight years of trying to find an employer who would keep her on in spite of her inability to remember even the simplest things.

As she grew older and more aware of her mental problem, Alison, usually in the company of her mother, sought advice from every medical and health source they could think of.

Although her memory was almost non-existent, her reasoning ability was as good as ever. It was just that having reasoned things out she could not later recall the conclusions she had come to.

Alison very quickly learned the only way to stay on course was to write herself an endless succession of notes.

The one bright spot in an other wise agonizing life was a job with the Coca Cola factory in Upper Hutt under the supervision of factory manager Pat West. In Mr. West, Alison found an employer willing to give her every chance. At last she had steady employment.

Her job was to operate a machine which performed a single repetitive task. Unexciting, certainly, but it was a job. Alison managed to keep the machine going by way of self-written notes which reminded her what to do.

Alison was now 27 years old. She was living in a flat on her own. Her family had moved to Raumati Beach.

She had first moved with them, but missed her job at the Coca Cola factory so much, she eventually moved back to Upper Hutt after Pat West said she could have her job back again.

In spite of the steady job, life was a tedious business for Alison Money. She too often forgot such elementary things as putting water in a pot before putting it on the stove, or she would forget to turn off the heater before going to bed.

Her only way of overcoming these difficulties was by referring to notes telling her what had to be done at any given time of the day.

For anyone with a normal memory and average intelligence it is hard indeed to imagine life without a fully functioning memory.

Perhaps the most telling description of Alison's plight came during the hearing before the Commission of Inquiry when Mrs. Money told the commissioners from the witness stand that one of the saddest things about Alison's problem was she could not read a book.

"Alison could never remember where she was up to, and even if she started reading again at the right place, she would have forgotten what the story was about anyway," she testified.

Then came another event in Alison's life which was to prove to be as dramatic in terms of future consequences as had been her accident so many years before. She visited Dr. Walter Williams, a chiropractor with a clinic in Upper Hutt.

It was not through any recommendation of established medicine that she came to visit the one health profession which could well have saved her many years of misery. Alison went to a chiropractor in response to her mother's suggestion, a suggestion following a personal experience of chiropractic care which Mrs. Money had just previously enjoyed.

Before the idea of chiropractic care was put to her by her mother, Alison had never heard of chiropractic. In all those years no one among all the health people from whom she had sought help had mentioned the possibility of chiropractic care.

In spite of her mother's urging, it took Alison weeks of agonizing inner debate just to dredge up the courage to make an appointment.

She knew only too well that any such appointment would require her to go through the frightening trip from her Trentham flat to the local railway station, from there by train to Upper Hutt-just a few miles away - and from the Upper Hutt station to the chiropractor's clinic.

A simple journey for most. But for Alison, a truly daunting ordeal. But, with the use of the inevitable script of directions, make the trip she did. Alison, if nothing else, was not lacking in courage.

Back in her flat a few hours later, Alison telephoned her mother and amid tears of unrestrained joy told how she had found her way back from the chiropractor to her flat without once having referred to a note.

It was February, 1977. She was 27 years of age. For the first time in 16 years she could actually remember the time of day, which way was the way home, and her mother's telephone number.

The commissioners learned that on her first visit to Dr. Williams, the chiropractor had immediately discovered an obvious abnormality in the upper area of the spine, undoubtedly caused by the trauma of Alison's head striking the concrete footpath a decade and a half before.

Just one adjustment was all it took to relieve pressure on a nervous system that had been in trauma for so many years.

Many visits to Dr. William's chiropractic center were to follow. If lasting benefit was to result, chiropractic care would have to continue for some time, but that first visit had been to all intents and purposes a rebirth for Alison Money.

A long and happy association with the Mormon Church inspired a burning desire for Alison to visit Salt Lake City in the United States of America. Now that Alison had made such a dramatic recovery, she and her mother set about the task of saving sufficient funds to finance such a trip.

In due course, the funds were set aside and Alison spent eight weeks in the United States.

That Alison had been able to find her way around the Los Angeles airport, renowned throughout the world for its expanse of connecting corridors which fan out in a multitude of directions, and that she had been able to travel about the US on Greyhound buses, was put forward as proof positive of Alison's incredible memory recovery.

On top of all this, Alison had sufficient confidence in herself to stand before thousands of Mormons at a conference and relate to them her years of misery and the remarkable recovery that chiropractic care had brought about.

In her submission to the Commission of Inquiry, Mrs. Money concluded by writing, "The medical profession and the physiotherapists may gain if they agree to work alongside the chiropractor.

"My daughter's amazing progress is proof that a chiropractor can give help where other professions fail. My great regret is that my daughter was not advised to see a chiropractor years ago."

The commissioners agreed that the Alison Money story was yet another remarkable testimony to the worth of chiropractic and chose to highlight this particular case in their published report to the government.

The original publication of the Alison File was delayed for more than 12 months. After researching the commission's records, and making an appointment to call on the family, I was distressed to discover that much of the dramatic improvement reported to the Commission of Inquiry had given way to an equally dramatic deterioration over the post-commission years.

On the day of my visit, Alison was clearly in a depressed state. Her mother said that Alison's periods of depression had become a regular way of life. For Mrs. Money, now a widow more or less restricted to looking after Alison, life was not all that pleasant either.

A refusal by medical people to recognize Alison's mental handicap as a major obstacle to obtaining regular employment meant that instead of being on an invalid benefit, Alison was forced to accept the unemployment benefit and its attendant requirement to constantly seek work. Each job interview, and the few trial periods she was offered, became periods of extreme stress.

As each job collapsed, the waiting for the next job interview required by law was almost as bad as the interview itself.

It was in this most unhealthy atmosphere of tension that Alison had begun the backward slide in mental health and well being.

Alison had returned to live with her mother after a change of supervisors at Coca Cola had turned that job into a misery for her. But the greatest blow to Alison's future came a year later when Alison's chiropractic care came to an end with the departure to Australia of the one and only chiropractor in the district.

When I called to interview the Moneys for this story, some four years had elapsed from the time of Dr. William's departure. In the meantime, another chiropractor was again practicing in the district.

I persuaded Alison to make an appointment and try chiropractic care, on a continuing basis, once again.

Although Alison's rapid improvement up to the time of the Commission of Inquiry had been yet another truly wonderful example of chiropractic in action, the interruption of that care for so many years had clearly taken its toll.

I felt I could not then in all conscience present the Alison File as yet another chronicle of chiropractic success. I therefore delayed publication to allow the restarted chiropractic program to produce what I fully believed would be the inevitable result.

And so it did.

When I telephoned Mrs. Money a year later, she reported that Alison was visiting Dr. Phelps on a continuing basis and as a result, Alison had again regained much of her memory.

The periods of depression had disappeared altogether.

Among other things, I saw she could again sit at the piano and play her favorite pieces from beginning to end without referring to sheet music. Alison had been learning to play the piano for about a year before the school ground accident put an end to that pleasure.

Alison at last had been referred to a medical specialist who immediately reported to the authorities that her mental problem was such that she should be on an invalid benefit- as clearly she should have been all along.

Perhaps she may never fully regain her memory function, but there was no doubting the benefits chiropractic care had once again brought to Alison. The dramatic change I personally witnessed during that second visit was as much an inspiration to me as had it been my own chiropractic experience.

But the most marvelous development of all was the discovery that Alison was engaged to be married.

It was definitely time for the Alison File to be published.

"I Need Never Have Retired"

In New Zealand, the job of Minister of Education is probably the least popular of the nation's cabinet posts. It is practically impossible for a Minister of Education to simultaneously earn the popular support of teachers, parents, and school boards.

Nevertheless, one man who did the seemingly impossible was the Minister of Education from 1963 to 1969, the honourable Arthur E. Kinsella. At age 52, after 15 years as Hauraki's electorate representative in New Zealand's House of Parliament, Kinsella was riding high on the crest of a wave of popularity and respect for the manner in which he was handling the most difficult portfolio.

In April, 1969, he was about to complete nine years as a cabinet minister. In government ranking, he was No. 3 and with an election coming up that year he was fully confident of another successful three-year term in the service of his country.

At 8:30 on the morning of April 24, 1969, Kinsella was relaxed and confident as he drove from Masterton to Palmerston North's Massey College where he was to appear as the main speaker in an education seminar.

And then tragedy struck. As he approached the northern end of the Manawatu Gorge, the axle of his state-owned ministerial car fractured, causing the right hand back wheel to fall away from its mounting. The car veered violently off the road and crashed into a power pole, ripping out the entire driver's side of the car in the process.

When the car eventually came to rest on its side, Kinsella, suffering from multiple injuries, was mercifully unconscious. He remembers little of the next few hours.

Ten years later, he was, however, able to testify to the chiropractic inquiry commissioners that he had ended up in the Palmerston North Hospital where his right leg had been encased in plaster to aid the healing process of a multiple fracture.

But, for some reason unknown to the patient, only cursory attention was given to the possibility of chest and internal injuries and none at all to the possibility of back injuries.

On the day after entering the hospital, he was discharged. Kinsella, still suffering considerable pain, found himself back in his Wellington ministerial residence.

That night as the result of intense pain and extreme discomfort, an ambulance was called by a hastily summoned local medical doctor. In the Wellington Hospital, surgeons discovered multiple internal injuries, including a crushed chest, diaphragm injuries and a ruptured spleen, all requiring urgent surgery.

Even so, no X-rays were taken to check on possible spinal damage. In fact Kinsella's complaints of severe back and neck pain were attributed by the medical experts to the internal injuries and would disappear after the crisis therapy of surgical intervention.

During hospitalization, the persisting back and neck pains were suppressed by drugs. After discharge, the still suffering patient was placed on a physiotherapy program under strict medical supervision.

In spite of the best attention medical science could offer, in the form of four-times-a-week physiotherapy sessions for a period of no less than six months, Kinsella's condition, in so far as mobility was concerned, deteriorated.

During this period, the provision of painkiller drugs and crutches enabled the patient to return to his parliamentary executive duties. However, as the nomination deadline for the November triennial parliamentary elections drew near, his condition continued to deteriorate. It inevitably became obvious Kinsella would be unable to stand the pace of an election campaign, let alone contribute to a successful outcome from the government's point of view.

He therefore approached the Prime Minister of the day and out of fairness to his constituents and to his party as a whole, tendered his resignation.

Thus an outstanding political career came to a calamitous end. Later, it was dramatically revealed if the correct medical advice and therapy had been given, resignation need never have been considered.

The official announcement to the country that Kinsella would no longer be available on the national political scene inspired a most uncharacteristic tide of editorial comment from the nation's leading newspapers.

Without exception, these hard-nosed newspaper professionals praised the outstanding abilities of the retiring cabinet minister. All expressed regret at his enforced departure. No education minister before or since has earned such high praise from the news media, the education profession, or the public at large.

At no time did Kinsella's numerous medical advisers consider the possibility of chiropractic advice or attention. In the medical world, such a thought would have amounted to virtual heresy.

The evidence given under oath to the Commission of Inquiry revealed that had a chiropractor been called in during the post-accident examination stage, the whole episode would have been but a temporary inconvenience in the onward progress of Kinsella's ministerial duties.

Painful, certainly. Nevertheless, nothing more nor less than a short-term set-back. If only. If. If. If...

But in 1969, the prejudice of the New Zealand medical fraternity to the science, art and philosophy of chiropractic was at its most virulent. There was even an official New Zealand Medical Association ethic that categorically and specifically forbade medical doctors to call in or refer to a chiropractor. Any medical doctor who disobeyed this edict was liable to severe disciplinary action.

Since the Commission of Inquiry, the Medical Association has been forced to remove this obnoxious ethic - after all, it flew in the face of legislative recognition of chiropractic. Even in 1996, there is a lingering antipathy to chiropractic by many in the medical profession.

Ironically, accident victim, Kinsella himself, contributed to this discriminatory state of affairs.

In the early 1950's, as a backbench member of a parliamentary investigative committee into the desirability or otherwise of giving chiropractors official recognition by way of statutory registration, Kinsella in fact, voted against such a proposal. (In 1960, legislation was enacted to register and thus officially recognize chiropractic.)

In 1979, he enhanced his credibility as a witness before the New Zealand Commission of Inquiry into Chiropractic by voluntarily revealing this earlier error of judgement.

It was to be almost two years from the time of the accident before chiropractic care was to restore the integrity of his spine, the source of Kinsella's continuing disability.

About a year before Chiropractic was to help the problem, Kinsella consulted an Auckland-based orthopedic specialist.

At that time, his leg condition was steadily deteriorating. He was suffering from continuing severe back pain, a chronic blurring of eyesight and severely restricted head and neck movement.

The specialist diagnosed an arthritic condition in the injured leg and in the right shoulder. He prescribed a continuation of painkiller drugs along with a further extensive medically-supervised physiotherapy program.

Neither course of action proved to be effective.

The first positive steps towards achieving total recovery were taken by executive committee members of the Royal Corps of NZ Engineers, of which Kinsella was a member by virtue of his World War II service.

His friends in the corps became increasingly concerned about the continual deterioration of the ex-cabinet minister's physical condition.

Their solution was to persuade Kinsella to visit a chiropractor.

By now Kinsella was experiencing extreme difficulty in walking, and then only with the aid of walking sticks. With increasing regularity he was prone to suddenly collapse in the street.

It was becoming apparent that for his own safety confinement to a wheelchair was not far distant.

In spite of all this, Kinsella would not be persuaded to place his case in the hands of a chiropractor. His decision was influenced by his memory of the "evidence" that had come before the parliamentary investigating committee many years before.

In the end, the corps members made an appointment without Kinsella's knowledge and virtually deposited him at the door of a chiropractic clinic.

The visit to the Auckland-based chiropractor, Dr. L. Duggan, was to prove to be the arresting and turning point in Kinsella's downward slide. After a thorough and comprehensive examination, using the considerable skills of the chiropractic profession, Dr. Duggan discovered serious dysfunction of a number of vertabrae in the neck region and at the base of the spine.

Kinsella testified at the commission hearing he had been shown two sets of X-rays.

"Even to the untrained eye, it was fairly obvious what the problem was. There was a definite curvature there. And a displacement. You could see it with the naked eye. It was clear even to an untrained person such as myself," he said.

Obviously, these aberrations were either caused or aggravated by the earlier car accident. In the intervening period considerable inflammation of the affected areas had occurred, along with a pronounced tilt in the pelvis which consequently threw most of the weight of the body onto the accident-weakened leg.

Kinsella testified to the astonished commissioners that Dr. Duggan had found no evidence of debilitating arthritis.

Commissioner Dr. Bruce Penfold, A Christchurch professor of chemistry, queried Kinsella: "You say in your submission that the chiropractor, after he had X-rayed you, did not detect any arthritic condition."

Kinsella: "No significant arthritic condition. He found there was some wearing of the joints and some slight indication of arthritis, but not enough to cause trouble."

Dr. Penfold: "Yet it was on the basis, presumably, of the X-ray from the medical specialist that the arthritic condition had been diagnosed."

Kinsella: "I had not been X-rayed at all by the medical profession, other than in connection with the leg fractures."

Later, in their official report to the government, the commissioners were to comment again and again on the apparent ignorance of the medical profession in respect to spinal examination.

And then Kinsella told the commission of the sequence of events leading to a complete recovery in an incredibly short space of time. Within one hour of Dr. Duggan administering the first vertebral adjustments to the upper and lower spine, Kinsella was able to walk freely, his vision cleared, the mobility in his neck improved remarkably and the pain in his legs became greatly relieved.

Kinsella was moved to say at the hearing: "It was not a miraculous treatment, but certainly it was miraculous that I became mobile within an hour."

During an interview with the author in 1984, Kinsella confirmed that there was no doubt in his mind that had he been referred to a chiropractor shortly after the accident, he would have been able to return to his ministerial duties within a very short time, fully mobile and well on the way to total recovery.

Resignation, he stressed, would never have become a consideration.

The commissioners closely questioned this witness about the lack of success by the medical profession over two years, followed by the remarkable success within one hour of chiropractic care.

Although witness after witness had told of similar recoveries, some within a matter of minutes of an adjustment by a chiropractor, the commissioners were still having trouble accepting the simplicity of chiropractic care, in comparison with the results achieved, especially when compared with the often lengthy therapy delivered by traditional medicine.

After more than 18 months of investigation and inquiry, the commissioners eventually accepted the truth and almost routine nature of such seemingly remarkable recoveries.

But Kinsella was only No. 24 in a list of more than 70 witnesses presenting similar evidence. When Kinsella gave his evidence, the underlying truth of chiropractic care had yet to be fully appreciated by the commissioners.

In Kinsella's case, it took only three weeks of adjustments for the total eradication of all signs of pain, swelling and disability.

To all intents and purposes, the patient was as fit and as well 21 days after receiving the first chiropractic adjustment as he had been immediately prior to the disastrous car accident.

Clearly, he should never have been required to abandon his political career.

In the litany of evidence presented to the commission concerning misguided drug and physiotherapy treatments prescribed by the medical profession, this was surely one of the saddest.

The recovery had come too late to save a brilliant career, a career that could have continued to exert so much positive influence in the lives of so many people.

On the other hand, the crucial chiropractic intervention did see a return to normal living, although away from public life. He again took up his teaching career, eventually taking charge of a 500-staff Technical Correspondence Institute in Wellington, a position he retained for almost a decade before retiring in 1983.

Although the Kinsella story is a remarkable testament to the effectiveness of chiropractic, there is still more to tell, for following full recovery, Kinsella had a habit of forgetting altogether he once came close to being crippled for life and that a reasonable degree of care was necessary to avoid recurring dysfunction of weakened spinal structures affected by the accident.

Consequently, he was inclined on occasions to lift items in a manner beyond the capabilities of those spinal segments.

One of the excuses for this seeming neglect was that Kinsella came to have an abiding faith in the ability of chiropractors to put matters right should they go wrong.

On at least three different occasions, it took what amounted to virtual emergency care administered by various chiropractors to restore his mobility.

On one occasion, for instance, over-exertion on his part resulted in a dysfunction of such severity that he was rendered completely immobile, more or less cast on his back and unable to move.

A member of his staff was called in to provide transport. After much painstaking and painful maneuvering, he was placed in the staff person's car and taken to the chiropractic clinic.

It took two people to carry him into the clinic. Later, his good Samaritan staff member was staggered to witness Kinsella walking out of the clinic as if nothing had ever happened.

Kinsella testified that on each and every occasion he had called on the chiropractic profession to provide urgent care, it had been immediately forthcoming and on each and every occasion that care had been 100% effective.

At the conclusion of his evidence, Kinsella made the following submission:

"That chiropractic be recognized as a legitimate specialist health service. It is obvious that present medical services has a serious gap in their knowledge and training in this particular field in which chiropractors are expert."

Case Studies — Part 2

The following case studies were taken directly out of the Chiropractic in New Zealand Report published in 1979 by The Government Printer, Wellington, NZ. This is one of the most thorough and positive studies of chiropractic care on record. The 20-month study was conducted by a government commission.

The Case of Mr. S

Mr. S had a persistent back problem. Early in 1977 his back became quite painful and he developed pain in his leg as well. His condition was diagnosed medically as rheumatism but he subsequently had X-rays taken and the resulting diagnosis was "wear and tear." He was given physiotherapy for 2 weeks without improvement and then carried on with it for another 3 or 4 weeks while he was waiting for an appointment with a specialist. The specialist recommended another 3 or 4 weeks of physiotherapy, but again there was no improvement. Mr. S had reservations about going to a chiropractor but in August 1977 the pain became so bad that he pushed his scruples aside. He attended for chiropractic care daily for a few weeks. At once there was a marked improvement. He now goes to his chiropractor about every 6 weeks as a preventative measure. The pain has disappeared from his leg and he is now able to drive his car without any discomfort.

The Case of Mr. P

Mr. P, who is an auditor in his late fifties, suffered constant backache. He was unable to sit or stand for any length of time. He could not sleep properly. He had extensive medical treatment including X-rays, consultations with specialists, and physiotherapy. He had always regarded chiropractors as "quacks" but his wife went to one, on the advice of a friend, for severe loss of balance resulting from a fall. Her condition greatly improved and Mr. P decided to visit a chiropractor too. He told us after only one adjustment the relief was so great he felt it was like a "miracle." After the initial care, he now goes only on the few occasions when his back gives him minor trouble.

The Case of Mrs. E

Mrs. E, a sensible mature woman, suffered back and leg injuries when her horse slipped and fell while she was helping to draft cattle. She spent 10 days in the hospital, the principal treatment being water baths to reduce the swelling in her leg. She was discharged on crutches and then graduated to a walking-stick, and she could not sleep at night unless she elevated her leg with a pillow to get relief from pain in her lower back. All this was a problem for her, the more so because she had a family of young children. Her general practitioner put her on valium, she said to ease the pain, but it did not help. Finally she consulted a chiropractor and after a short course of care found the pain suddenly disappeared and she was able to walk normally. She told us every now and then when she was bumped by a farm animal or had some other minor accident her back played up, but she got immediate relief from chiropractic care. Apart from such minor and passing incidents she has had no further problems.

The Case of Mr. J

Mr J is a solicitor. He has had experience of personal injury claims for clients with back problems and he told us his clients had frequently been relieved from quite considerable pain even after a short course of chiropractic care. Mr. J's main evidence was, however, in relation to his own personal experience. He was on the Wahine when it foundered at the entrance of the Wellington Harbor. He suffered a back injury which was a matter of great concern to him during the following year. He was able to get out of bed only with great difficulty, and he was in considerable and continuous pain. He consulted medical practitioners who prescribed painkillers which were only of limited assistance to him. Finally he went to a chiropractor and as a result of the care he received he has had few problems with his back since. Mr J initially had chiropractic care every 2nd day for 6 or 8 days; then the care was reduced to once a week for 2 weeks; and then reduced again, until finally there was a consultation only at 6-monthly intervals.

The Case of Mr. R

Mr. R's experience of chiropractic took place many years ago, but his case is of interest. He is a farmer. Thirty years ago he suffered an injury to his back. Bone fusion surgery was prescribed. A few days before he was to enter the hospital a friend persuaded him to try a chiropractor. After a course of care the effects of his injury disappeared and for 20 years he has not required further chiropractic care. He is now 77 and is in excellent health. He still farms. He shears sheep and takes part in axemen's events at the local sports. Photographs were shown to us of Mr. R, vigorously competing as an axeman at the 1977 local sports.

The Case of Mrs. D

Mrs. D told us she was severely injured in a car accident at the age of 7. She had had medical treatment for years. She ended up with a stabilizing brace which she wore for about 10 years. Finally she saw a chiropractor. He X-rayed her and said he would do his best to help her but because the injury to her spine was of such long-standing nature, he could not guarantee complete success. After the first adjustment she walked out of his rooms without the brace and without pain. She was able, as she told us, "...to enjoy [a] healthy active pain-free body."

The Case of Matron P

The matron of a private hospital gave evidence before the Commission. She has had extensive hospital experience. Some years ago she had a neck problem that was medically diagnosed as a disc lesion. She was given cortisone injections and a neck collar was pre-scribed. She also underwent physiotherapy. None of these treatments improved her condition. Ultimately, as the result of a suggestion made by a medical practitioner she knew, she consulted a chiropractor. She made it a condition of consulting him that any X-ray he took should first be examined by her medical practitioner before any chiropractic care was undertaken. That was done, and she went in for chiropractic care. Her neck condition immediately improved: she told us she had "never looked back." As might be expected from her background, the witness was unemotional in speaking about her condition and its cure. She had at the start been predisposed against chiropractic by reason of her training, but her personal experience of it led her to see advan-tages in it, at least for her type of case. She felt chiropractic care had been the answer to her problem, for which no earlier treatment had been effective. Her case is therefore a typical one. It is mentioned because her position of authority in hospital management and her training makes her a particularly accurate and reliable witness.

The Case of Mr. F

Mr. F is a carrier, in business on his own account. His colleagues in the carrying trade persuaded him to try chiropractic care when he was suffering from a painful and nearly useless shoulder. He found the chiropractor professional, sympathetic, and realistic. X-rays were taken, carefully analyzed and after five brief sessions of care he was back to normal.

More recently he suffered from sciatica. His general practitioner referred him to an experienced physiotherapist but after three sessions of ultrasonic treatment Mr. F was no better and he turned to the chiropractor who had cared for him previously. The chiropractor quickly relieved his sciatica, which had not returned when Mr. F gave his evidence.

Mr. F saw chiropractic as being particularly valuable to the self-employed worker who cannot afford to take a leisurely cure. The main point he wanted to make was the rapid results obtainable from chiropractic care as opposed to orthodox treatment.

The Case of Mr. V

Mr. V has had a bad back since 1933. He was injured in a car accident. He is a civil engineer and the work he does requires him to be able to move around freely. For the first 10 years after his accident he spent long periods of time in bed and was at one time partially paralyzed. He was prescribed pain-relieving pills and several courses of physiotherapy but these did him little good. He eventually went to the chiropractor and benefited greatly.

He now goes on the average once a month. The purpose of the chiropractic care is mainly to keep him on his feet. It is a case where he would not need to visit the chiropractor so frequently if the work he did demanded less strain on his back, but his career requires this kind of work and he also likes to keep active around the house. So he undergoes chiropractic care whenever he thinks he needs it as part of the cost of staying active.

Mr. V improved to the stage where 4 years ago he was able to build his own house. This is an example of a case where regular chiropractic care was able to keep an active man both in his career and doing work which he enjoys and which would otherwise be impossible.

The Case of Mr. G

Mr. G was immobilized by a back injury in 1970. His medical adviser told him he would need to be in the hospital and probably in traction for some weeks. His wife called in a chiropractor who cared for him and within 2 weeks he was back to normal.

This was the effect of this witness's formal submission, but in the course of giving oral evidence, he told us about a completely different matter affecting his wife. He told us he and his wife had found it impossible during some 6 years of marriage to have a child. They had undergone intensive physical and gynecological tests and were told there was nothing wrong. They adopted two children over a period. Mrs. G was sometime afterward persuaded by a friend to consult a chiropractor about her infertility. She was apprehensive. Her husband went with her for the consultation. The chiropractor examined her and found what her husband described as a misplaced vertebra. The chiropractor gave Mrs. G one adjustment. Shortly after that she became pregnant.

This evidence was given quite spontaneously when Mr. G was asked by the Commission if he felt the fixing of back pain was the limit of what a chiropractor normally does. Mr. G then told us about his wife's experience.

The Case of Mr. H

Mr. H, who was retired and in his seventies, had been seriously hurt in a motor accident. His head had been injured in some way which he was unable to specify, but the result of the injury was that he suffered extreme discomfort if he tried to lie on the side that had suffered the damage. At an earlier time of his life he had suffered from asthma which had, however, naturally remitted. But it came on again when he was in his sixties. He took prescribed medication for his asthma.

Mr. H gave us a very refreshing, direct, and dramatic account of his consultation with the chiropractor. He told the chiropractor on no account to do anything that would affect his head. However, the chiropractor did so. Mr. H protested forcibly and pungently but later found to his amazement he had lost both the unpleasant consequences of his head injury and also his asthma. He told us this: "Anyway on the Monday he went over me and he said, "Mr. H, in my opinion, in a few days you will be quite alright." To my astonishment I have been quite alright since."

The Case of Mrs. M

About 12 months ago Mrs M was in a car accident and suffered a whiplash injury which affected her neck. After hospital and physiotherapy treatment for 2 weeks she was still in severe pain and she went to her chiropractor and was cared for quickly and successfully.

Mrs. M also suffered from high blood pressure, water retention (oedema), and headaches. When she visited the chiropractor concerning her neck problem she was asked what medication she was on. She told the chiropractor about her blood pressure, a condition from which she had suffered for over 15 years, her water retention problem and her headaches. The chiropractor told her that after a course of chiropractic care her blood pressure could be expected to go down so she would not have to take medication continually, and her water retention would improve. Mrs. M told us that although she had confidence in the chiropractor's ability to fix her neck she was very doubtful about his capacity to relieve the other conditions. She said this in her formal submission: "To my surprise, and great satisfaction, everything he has told me has transpired. My blood pressure is now normal, (I now take no blood pressure tablets) and my water retention has improved 75%. (I now take tablets about once weekly instead of every day)...I should like to mention my headaches have almost completely disappeared."

Mrs. M was sensible enough to have her blood pressure and water retention conditions monitored by her regular medical practitioner. In cross-examination she told us her doctor was quite surprised her blood pressure had reverted to normal.

This was one of the occasions on which the Medical Association applied for and was granted leave to obtain an expert medical opinion. Mrs. M consented to her medical records being examined, and a medical expert was appointed to examine them.

We have received his report, which is limited to the question of blood pressure. The records of Mrs. M's own doctor show during 1970 Mrs. M's blood pressure fluctuated between 170/120 and 120/190 but was on most occasions at a level indicating moderate hypertension. There is only one reading recorded in 1971 (126/104), and then there is a gap in the readings until April 1976 (150/106). The readings in May, July and August 1976 indicate moderate to mild hypertension, and "normal" readings are recorded in November and December 1976, and January 1977. On 9 May 1977 the reading shows a mild degree of hypertension (140/100); similarly on 30 May 1977. On 15 September 1977 a normal reading is recorded, as it is on either 12 December 1977 or 12 February 1978 (the date is not clear from the report). The reading had returned to mild (135/95) on 1 June 1978 and on 13 October 1978 (140/96), the last reading we have.

The records show that until late 1977 Mrs. M was on blood pressure lowering drugs. Declinax was stopped in either December 1977 or February 1978, and on 1 June 1978 the record reads "Tenuate Dospan prescribed, taking Lasix on and off." No prescription is recorded against the entry of 13 October 1978. (It should be noted Mrs. M's formal submission to the Commission is dated 24 May 1978, and she presented it orally on 7 August 1978.)

The medical expert's conclusion was there is no justification for the claim the chiropractic treatment returned Mrs. M's blood pressure to normal. He reports the normal readings achieved on and after 15 September 1977 could have been due to the antihypertensive medication, other factors, or to the variable nature of the mild hypertension itself. Because no readings were taken before Mrs. M was put on antihypertensive medication, it cannot be demonstrated either Mrs. M's normal readings were achieved by the antihypertensive medication.

The records are consistent with what Mrs. M told us. She told us she had been taking antihypertensive medication for 15 years. She said her blood pressure had always been "slightly above what was considered to be normal, but not excessively when I was taking medication" (Transcript, p. 871).

As to the water retention problem, Mrs. M said "if I did not take my water retention tablets prior to my care with [the chiropractor], my ankles would swell up badly and it was noticeable, and my weight would increase rapidly also because of fluid, and I had to take these tablets every day in order to keep it under control. Now I find I am able to keep it under control with tablets only once or twice a week" (Transcript, p. 872).

It seems clear by late 1977 or early 1978 Mrs. M's doctor took the view the ganglion-blocking agent (Declinax) as medication for hypertension was no longer required. Mrs. M's intake of the rapidly acting diuretic agent (Lasix) had been reduced by June 1978, when medication specifically designed to reduce obesity by suppressing appetite was prescribed (Tenuate Dospan). That appears to be consistent with what Mrs. M told us.

Naturally in the circumstances no firm conclusion can be drawn either on whether the prescribed medication in fact had any effect on Mrs. M's hypertension, or on whether the chiropractic care had any effect on it. The Commission is left with facts and probabilities.

The facts are before Mrs. M had chiropractic care she was demonstrated to have mild to moderate hypertension and in the year prior to chiropractic care was being medicated by two drugs, one a quick-acting diuretic, and the other a hypotensive agent which acts by selectively blocking transmission in the post-ganglionic adrenergic nerves. After her chiropractic care her blood pressure dropped back to normal, although it later increased to a mild degree, she was taken off the ganglion-blocking agent, and her intake of the diuretic agent reduced.

The probabilities are the chiropractic care did have the effect both of relieving her hypertension and reducing her dependency on medication, although naturally other possibilities cannot be ruled out.

The Case of Mr. R's Small Boy

Mr. R was a chiropractic patient who had suffered from a serious back problem for which he had obtained relief by chiropractic treatment.

One day Mr. R told his chiropractor he was concerned about the condition of his little boy, not quite 2 years old, who was an asthmatic. The child had been taken to a specialist and was under medical care, but he seemed to be getting worse. As Mr. R testified (Submission 36, p. 4):

By this time my son had developed a constant wheeze and was losing weight due to his inability to eat the right quantity of food, plus he was finding it very difficult to sleep at night due to the wheezing and shortness of breath.

And under very intensive cross-examination Mr. R spoke of his son "surging, gasping for breath," and he and his wife had to take it in turns sitting with the little boy throughout the night in case the child woke up and needed attention and comforting.

The chiropractor suggested Mr. R bring the child in for examination. He did not promise a cure. Mr. and Mrs. R took the little boy in. The chiropractor examined him, suggested the child might have had a fall at some time (which was the case) and adjusted the child's neck.

Immediately there was a dramatic improvement. Mr. R described it, in a spontaneous answer under cross-examination, as "miraculous." "We didn't even get out of the waiting room and his constant wheeze, which was pretty bad, had almost disappeared." Some months later, and after some further chiropractic adjustments, the little boy's asthmatic symptoms had completely gone. On the night of the first treatment the child had his first uninterrupted sleep for some considerable time.

As we have said, Mr. R was intensively cross-examined, and we therefore had a full opportunity to assess what weight we could place on his evidence. The Commission was most impressed with him. It was clear his son's instant response to the chiropractic care had left a deep impression on him. He did not expect any particular result, and that is why he spontaneously described the result as "miraculous." He was reliving the moment as he told us that.

It was put to Mr. R in cross-examination that his son's asthmatic condition could have relieved itself naturally, and (in effect) that chiropractic care had nothing to do with it. Mr. R rejected that suggestion and so do we: we cannot accept that within minutes of the chiropractic care the little boy's asthmatic symptoms remitted themselves purely by coincidence. We are driven to find the major relief the child experienced within that short time was a direct result of the chiropractic care he received.

The Case of Mrs. D's Daughter

Mrs. D told us of chiropractic relief which had been given to her young daughter.

Her daughter suffered from impaired hearing. Mrs. D and her husband took her to an ear, nose, and throat specialist. The specialist thoroughly examined her and recommended surgery. Mrs. D was reluctant to agree to this course, and thought that chiropractic should at least be tried. Mrs. D had been to a chiropractor for a back complaint. She and her husband took the child to the chiropractor who examined her and adjusted her spine in the area of the neck.

Much to Mr. and Mrs. D's surprise, the child was able to hear a whisper from across the room the following day. In Mrs. D's words, recalling the child's previous condition, "that to me was miraculous."

They took the child back to the ear, nose, and throat specialist. The specialist tested the child. He found, to his surprise, that her hearing had improved to a level of 100/98. That was a remarkable change. Her hearing had become normal. He asked what the parents had been doing. They told him they had taken the child to the chiropractor and his response, according to Mrs. D was "Of course if you are going to do this sort of thing you might get temporary relief but you will have her back here within 6 months."

Mrs. D told us the prediction had fortunately proved incorrect. Mrs. D went on to say that her daughter "is now trained as a nurse and she has no problem. In fact, her hearing is a little bit too good sometimes."

This case provides an interesting modern parallel with the first recorded chiropractic adjustment by Daniel David Palmer which is said to have affected a cure of deafness. It is unfortunate it was not possible to inquire into this particular case further by inviting the specialist and the chiropractor to give evidence before us. However, we have no reason to think, from seeing and hearing Mrs. D on the witness stand, that she was giving us other than an accurate and unemotional report.

Case Studies — Part 3

CASE STUDY

One day, about two years ago, the opportunity arose to provide chiropractic to 20 multi-handicapped, abused, abandoned, born addicted children. These were children with severe congenital, genetic and acquired afflictions.

I realized if I were to show how wonderful chiropractic can be, then it must be subjected to the hard core medical failures. The ones where no placebo effect is possible.

This group included children born to crack, alcohol and pill addicts, either one or all. Children shaken until blind, epileptic, and retarded. Beaten with hammers and thrown against walls. Sexually molested and abused until autistic. Anencephalic and hydrocephalics. Mentally retarded, cerebral palsy, dwarfism, blind, deaf, sickle cell anemia, herpes, born with internal organs outside, and other type afflictions associated with being shut away and drugged into submission, such as chronic infections, treated with antibiotics until weeping sores developed from fungal and other dermal problems. This home was full of disease and hopelessness. I was overwhelmed. Where do I start? What should I do?

I decided to make a commitment to begin adjusting them for as long as I remain in Miami, at least once a week.

The first day to adjust them arrived. The nurse administrator and assistant went around with me and held each baby while I palpated according to the teachings I was fortunate enough to receive from Dr. Larry Webster. Minimal pressure or force was utilized at each level of involvement until all vertebra were checked.

All the children were receptive and not one cried, sensing what was being done was natural, whether cognitively aware or not.

On my next visit it was reported one six-year old girl with epilepsy was having less severe and less often seizures. On my third visit, after two weeks, a four year old who could not walk or talk, was starting to walk (by four weeks he was running). He also was dwarfic, (looking like a two-year old). Within one year, he was speaking to age, and had grown to normal height.

Soon, everyone noticed the coughs, runny noses and fevers were gone! The weeping scalp and skin sores had healed. The herpes had cleared. The scissoring of the cerebral palsy were gone. Appetites were better, behavior was improved and the drooling stopped. The episodes of sickle cell diminished and cleared quicker. The congenital torticollis had eased considerably. The autistic girl stopped circling and singing and began to speak and act appropriately.

Miracles had appeared before our very eyes with simple, accurately applied pressure of 5 ounces to the spine. Here we see how far reaching the effects of removing subluxations with chiropractic can be to the health of the most afflicted children. Imagine how healthy the average loved and nurtured child from a caring biological family can be.

— Doctor of Chiropractic

CASE STUDY

Breana came into my office for examination and treatment of October of 1996. She had a history of intermittent vomitting, loss of sleep, diahrea, lethargy and the child would awaken and scream, not cry, but scream "MOM!" The mother said that Breana's tone of voice in the morning was definitely not that of the typical crying fit but that it was similar to some type of painful distress. The mother had taken Breana to the pediatrician on a number of occasions receiving the usual prescription of antibiotics with no improvements in Breana's well being. Breana weighed 16 pounds at 20 months while her identical twin sister weighed 20 pounds and was quite active. (An identical twin sister developing in a different way early in life. This is the difference between a child with subluxations, which repress expression of life and growth and development, versus a child without subluxations.) The mother states that her two daughters eventually became as different as night and day in their temperments and activity levels. Upon examining Breana's cervical spine, I palpated and found subluxations at C5 on the left and C1-C3 on the right. I questioned the mother if Breana had sustained any recent trauma or if she had been difficult to deliver. The mother said, "No." I adjusted Breana's cervical spine on Friday evening. The following Monday I received a call from Breana's mother stating that Breana is a totally different child. She gained two-and-a-half pounds over the weekend and she is no longer experiencing the aforementioned symptoms. "Thank you for giving me my child back," she stated.

— Doctor of Chiropractic

CASE STUDY

Years ago I had an 8 year-old boy that was classed as Mental Retarded. He was supposed to never evolve above the age of 3. He came in for care and we started adjusting him. He was also a mute. He was in the office one day and I walked into the reception room and all of the sudden he was pointing to pictures and asking, "what's that and what's that." I looked at his mother and said, "he has now awakened to a new world." After another month of adjusting, we sent him back for an IQ evaluation. His IQ was 44 when he first came to see me. He went back for an evaluation and he was evaluated at 88. The people who did the IQ evaluation wanted to know what had made this possible. The next month they enrolled him into a regular school. This is the same boy who was never supposed to evolve past the age of 3.

— Doctor of Chiropractic

CASE STUDY

Many newborns and infants are vomiting up to 15 times a day and stop almost immediately after a few adjustments. Colicky babies who scream constantly, miraculously stop once the nerve interference is gently removed and kids with ear infections get better when nerve flow is improved. The conditions that respond to chiropractic care are unlimited - from bedwetting to learning problems. We had a 12 month old who couldn't crawl and after one hip adjustment ran in the door to greet us on the next visit. This week I saw a baby who had the right side of her face compressed during the birth process. At 8 weeks old, one side of her head was 2 1/2" wider than the other. After using the Webster cranial technique, the measurements were almost even and have stayed that way since. It is truly a miracle when infants and children have their life force turned on.

— Doctor of Chiropractic

CASE STUDY — 5 INDIVIDUALS

CASE STUDY #1 (Boy, age 3)

Experiencing 30-50 petit mal (epileptic) seizures daily since birth. The child was on the usual seizure medications with negative results. The parents brought the child in for chiropractic care, stating: "This is the last resort." After six weeks of care, the seizures diminished to two per day. Needless to say, the parents were overjoyed.

CASE STUDY #2 (Twin boys, age 11)

Both with asthma, both experiencing vomiting daily for a period of five months. Both boys had a weight loss of 15 pounds giving them a gaunt and emaciated appearance. During this period, the mother had taken them to various doctors, including neurologists, psychiatrists, etc. to no avail. After the second adjustment, the asthma abated and after the third adjustment, the vomiting stopped. The boys also had not attended a full day of school in those five months but became able to do so. Their energy level increased and weight gain came about with an overall improvement in health.

CASE STUDY #3 (Boys, [Not related] ages 11 months and four years)

Both with Down's Syndrome. The younger one - severe, weighing seven pounds, with no gain since birth - was unable to retain any nourishment. After his first adjustment, he took four ounces of milk and gained two pounds in the following two weeks. Parents were amazed... The older one had usual Down's Syndrome symptoms and was unable to walk, talk or feed himself. After six months of care, he could dress himself, and was speaking more words. Parents had to fence in the yard because he was running all over the neighborhood. At age five-and-a-half (and still under care) he can feed himself and uses the bathroom by himself.

CASE STUDY #4 (Girl, age 5)

Classed as Mentally Retarded with an evaluated IQ of 46. She was adjusted for 30 days. Re-evaluated by the same center, she showed an IQ of 84. The child is now in the second grade leading a normal life.

CASE STUDY #5 (Boy, age 10)

Hyperactive, with an extremely limited span of concentration. After one-and-a-half months of care, there was a complete change of personality and the boy became a straight-A student.

— Doctor of Chiropractic

CASE STUDY

A six year old boy with nightly nocturnal enuresis, attention deficit disorder and toe walking found a chiropractor for chiropractic care. He walked with his heels 4 inches above the ground. The medical specialist recommended that both Achilles' tendons be cut and both ankles be broken to achieve normal posture and gait.

Chiropractic findings included subluxation of atlas, occiput, sacrum and pelvis (INEX). He had a mild scoliosis in the dorsal and lumbar regions. In addition, both tali and tibia/fibular articulations were misaligned. Foot dorsiflexion was absent bilaterally.

After 4 weeks of care, both heels dropped 2 inches and the bedwetting frequency decreased to 2-3 times per week. His doctor could not believe how chiropractic care made such a change and wants to meet the chiropractor. "One doctor at a time."

— Doctor of Chiropractic

CASE STUDY

A six week old baby with colic could not sleep for more than one hour at a time and could not hold food down. She was examined and diagnosed with a subluxation of the atlas. Also, there was a positive Fencer's reflex. After the first adjustment, the infant fell asleep before leaving the office and slept for 8 hours straight. There was a weight gain of 2 pounds in one week.

The child was seen 3 times per week for 2 months and then was reduced to once a week for maintenance. Adjustments consisted of light toggle and sustained pressure on the atlas. The colic symptoms have never returned.

— Doctor of Chiropractic

CASE STUDY

A seven year old girl had severe skin lesions covering much of her body "from her neck to her ankles." She was diagnosed at age 4 and had been treated with cortisone creams with no success. Past history revealed a forceps delivery.

Her parents took her to a chiropractor. Chiropractic analysis including x-rays and palpation revealed rotation of C2 (BR) and muscle spasms in the cervical spine with fixation of C1-C2. She was checked and adjusted 2 times per week. Within 4 weeks she was 90-95% better. She continued care for 2 more months.

— Doctor of Chiropractic

CASE STUDY

A four year old boy with headaches, vomiting, nasal drip and decreased appetite was diagnosed with orbital sinusitis. He was being treated with large doses of antibiotics. Past history revealed a fall on his head at the age of two from a height of 4 feet.

He was brought to a chiropractor. Chiropractic analysis revealed a left cervical rotation with retrolysthesis and rotation of C2. He also had fixation at the level of C2. He was seen 2 times per week for six months. The results were excellent. No more headaches, vomiting or nasal drip. In addition, his attitude and appetite dramatically improved.

— Doctor of Chiropractic

CASE STUDY

A five year old boy fell from his bike and within one week had symptoms of Bell's Palsy. The boy was unable to close his right eye or wrinkle his brow. He was brought to a neurologist who told the parents it would be 4 or 5 months recovery time.

The child was taken to a chiropractor for chiropractic care. Upon examination, the child was found to have a right lateral atlas with restriction in both right lateral flexion and right rotation. The patient was adjusted 1 time per week for three weeks at which time the symptoms had improved 90%. He has been under wellness care ever since.

— Doctor of Chiropractic

CASE STUDY

A 3 month old female infant was refusing to breastfeed for several days. A few days prior, her head had been whipped backward while being picked up by her older brother.

She was brought into a chiropractor's office. Upon examination, subluxation was found at the levels of Occiput, C2 and C3. After one adjustment, the infant began nursing, but only on one side. She was nursing normally on both sides after her second adjustment the following day. She continued for 6-8 more visits and is now receiving wellness care.

— Doctor of Chiropractic

CASE STUDY

One child could not crawl or talk and had severe muscle contractures, especially in his legs, prior to being brought in for chiropractic care. He was a refugee from one of the war zones in Croatia. B.E.S.T. and Diversified techniques were utilized by the chiropractor. By the time the family returned to their home area, the child had crawled, was talking and starting to walk. This was after about one year of care. I initially saw him 3 times per week and then slowly reduced it to 1 time every two weeks.

— Doctor of Chiropractic

CASE STUDY

A seven year old girl, Martina, was diagnosed with autism. When she first started coming in for chiropractic care about 14 months ago, the only thing she noticed was the light. She would not acknowledge anyone or respond to any type of stimulus. She showed almost no improvement for about 3 months.

Then one day when I came in and greeted her, she turned and looked me straight in the face. Her mother said something and she looked at her. Last week when they were in, her parents said she is now starting to point to her mouth and indicate when she is hungry. I can't tell you what a joy it is to have a child like this start to come into our world. I know that one of these days she will talk to us. She just had her eighth birthday.

— Doctor of Chiropractic

CASE STUDY — 6 INDIVIDUALS

Female, age 10. The child had poor grades due to lack of focus on homework and parental supervision was needed to complete homework. After three months of care she received most improved student award for bringing grades of an F and a D to an A and a B.

Male, age 13. History included traumatic birth (cord wrapped around neck) and did not crawl as a young child. After four weeks of care (including learning to cross crawl) he improved his grades from four F's to a B, D and notable improvements in the remaining two classes.

Male, age 12. He was run over by a car while riding a skateboard at age 5. He exhibited severe discipline problems at school with school suspension several times due to inappropriate behavior. He was failing all of his classes when he began chiropractic care. There has been little behavior improvement but grades have improved to a B, 3 C's and two D's.

Male, age 15. His birth was a C-section. He tested positive for food allergies and had severe hand tremors. After one week of care, parents and patient noticed hand tremors diminished. After five months of care, grades improved to 3 A's, 2 B's and 1 C (in personal fitness).

Female, age 15. X-rays revealed a severely reversed cervical curve. She was unable to allow anyone to touch her neck. In addition, she has a hypersensitivity to sounds. This is exhibited by the patient reflexively drawing her arms up to her neck with wrists flexed in a Palsy-like fashion. After two months of care, she noted she was able to get her hair washed at the hairdresser. Sounds were not as irritating to her anymore.

Male, age 9. He had a lack of focus at school and was a bed-wetter. After two months of care, his grades improved two letter grades. When his mother discontinued his care for a month, his grades dropped. He is back under care and grades are steadily improving. His focus has not improved to date.

— Doctor of Chiropractic

CASE STUDY

On July 10, 1995, a mother was referred for chiropractic care for her 7-year-old daughter. The presenting complaints were asthma and enuresis.

The birth of the child was a Ceserean type. As a child, she was inoculated with one Polio shot at age 2 and one Diphtheria/Tetanus shot. At the age of 2, she had the chicken pox and the flu. At the age of 3, asthma began to occur, along with many colds and flu's. The asthma got worse with age. The asthma required one hospitalization for 3 days and a series of trips to the emergency room due to the severe effects of the asthmatic attacks. Medication included Intal twice daily, Proventil at onset of an episode, and the constant company of a nebulizer for the exacerbated episodes when the breathing was labored or became a crisis. The mother reports her daughter would cough up a ball of phlegm following each episode. Also reported was the frequent amount of bloody noses she has experienced.

A thorough chiropractic examination with full spine films was taken and analyzed. Vertebral subluxations existed at C-2, T-5, T-12, the right Iliuma nd the second sacral tuberosity. Postural analysis showed a left head tilt, right high shoulder and left high ilium indicating the body was adapting to the stresses of the multiple subluxations.

The patient improved following the first adjustment and after the fifth adjustment, the asthma and bedwetting ceased. The stabilization of the VSC took 6 months at 3 times per week. Care was reduced to 2 times per week for 6 months and now the patient is checked once a week in the wellness phase to maintain the corrections of the VSC and wellness.

Today the patient is an extremely active child participating in all activities a young person enjoys. She continues to follow up with the advised wellness care allowing her body to heal itself as only it know how to do.

— Doctor of Chiropractic

CASE STUDY

A troubled mother was referred for chiropractic care concerning her 12-year-old son. Her son, since the age of 3, has had non-stop sinus infections every 2-3 months. The standard antibiotics, and occasionally the very potent ones, were used in an effort to control the infections. Previous surgeries included removal of the tonsils and adenoids at age 3. This latest bout was severe and surgery was mentioned to the mother as a possible resort.

Examination findings by postural analysis found a right high ear, left high posterior scapula, high and externally rotated left hip and anterior translation of the head. Differential temperature instrumentation noted C-2, C-7, T-3, T-5, T-8. Motion palpation found C-2, C-7, T-3, T-5, T-8 and right illium fixated.

Recommendations were made for adjustments at 4 times a week for the first 2 weeks, followed by 3 times a week for the next ten weeks to be changed as required and re-examined at the end of that time.

The parents chose to end the use of antibiotics and the patient was asymptomatic with the presenting complaint of sinus infections after the second visit. After 3 weeks into care, the cervical muscles are balancing out and the body posture is correcting to the point where the young patient is now carrying his head in an upright position. Both the patient and parents are aware of the quality of life that is returning as an apparent result of the chiropractic care. When the body loses its normal functioning nervous system and can no longer express life at its highest potential, the quality of life is always affected.

— Doctor of Chiropractic

CASE STUDY

Boy, age 14 months, with fluid in the ears was scheduled for implantation of tubes. He was adjusted 2 times at the atlas and axis area. The child was re-examined by his M.D., and surgery was cancelled.

— Doctor of Chiropractic

CASE STUDY

Boy, age 16 months, was scheduled to have cast to correct foot inversion. The pelvis was adjusted as an EX for a total of 6 times. Reevaluation by his pediatrician revealed complete correction and casting was cancelled.

— Doctor of Chiropractic

CASE STUDY

Female, age 3 years, appeared with severe torticolis with the head tilt to the left. Bracing had been recommended by medical doctors. The atlas was the segment adjusted with immediate correction occurring.

— Doctor of Chiropractic

CASE STUDY

Jonathan, Joel and Bryan, three little boys ages are 5, 7 & 10, all brought in with similar symptoms: constant congestion, inability to breathe, watery eyes, runny nose, wheezing, coughing and history of ear infections. All three were or had been on various medications ranging from antibiotics to bronchodilators to Prednisone.

As a chiropractor specializing in women's and children's health care, I would have to say at least 50% of all kids brought in for care present with the above symptoms. Most often by the time they get to me (I am a last resort), their mothers are desperate and willing to try anything. I just feel badly for the child, that they tried all the radical procedures first. Classically, a history will involve a difficult birth, either malpositioned or a long labor. Most of these children have also had several ear infections early in life.

Jonathan showed subluxations of the atlas, 74-75 area, and a right sacroiliac joint fixation. Joel: atlas and 74. And Bryan: atlas and 75- also had cranial faults.

The adjustments allowed the children to sleep better and get more rest. The subluxations were corrected and Bryan stabilized within 1 month (6-8 adjustments) and Joel within 1 1/2 months (8 adjustments). Jonathan went home after the 1st visit and showed immediate changes. I told the moms to keep track of any changes after the initial adjustment and to expect that the child may run a slight fever initially.

It's exciting to see children's little bodies respond almost instantly to the renewed nerve flow and vascular support that an adjustment provided. Due to less years of abuse, the little armies of defense attack viruses and bacteria without any help from us as long as there is no nerve interference.

— Doctor of Chiropractic

CASE STUDY

Two boys, ages 3 years and 9 months respectively. Both boys have been suffering from asthma since birth. They have been taking both inhalers and medication which did not help them sleep through the night without coughing or a shortness of breath. Their mother brought them in for chiropractic care and within 2 weeks (6 adjustments) their breathing was "normal" - meaning no coughing, wheezing, congestion, and both boys could sleep through the night. Both boys had a palpable muscle spasm along the right side, T4 - T8.

— Doctor of Chiropractic

CASE STUDY

A girl, age 14 1/2 , complained of headaches daily and a pain in her right hip. She was very active in school (cheerleading, jazz and ballet class, different school committees, etc.). Rotational malposition of cervical (C2 BL and C5 BR). The sacrum was adjusted Base Posterior on the right with left body rotation on the lumbar spine. Headaches disappeared after 2 days, hip pain was relieved in 4 adjustments.

— Doctor of Chiropractic

CASE STUDY

Bonnie is the mother of 5 children (all sickly and missing school every other day). The oldest, a girl, age 11, complained of headaches every day. The middle two girls, ages 5 & 7, both caught colds easily and were always sick. The 7-year-old also had vision problems and wears corrective lenses. The youngest two girls, age 2 & 3, had problems with their ears and also with chronic congestion. Bonnie has brought them in once a week for about two months. She realized nobody had missed school or complained about aches and pains in months. Chiropractic Works.

— Doctor of Chiropractic

CASE STUDY

A boy, age 18 months, was brought in by his mother for chiropractic care. The child was covered with exfoliative dermatitis, over 100% of his body. He had a fever of 102 degrees and his eyes were swollen closed. He looked like a bloated, swollen, red, moon-surfaced balloon.

A history revealed he was on a regimen of 10 medications, both oral and topical, for a week, with no improvement. The atlas and dorsal areas were adjusted and the parents decided to discontinue all medications. The child was brought back in the afternoon, and the parent stated the boy had slept calmly for 3 hours, for the first time in a week. His fever had dropped below 100 degrees, his eyes were wide open, and a clear patch had begun on his forehead.

After 2 weeks of daily adjustments, the skin was back to normal. Mind you, when I first saw him, I was speechless and in shock. I could not imagine what I might do. I ignored my fear and just adjusted the subluxations. I thought, "Let me do my duty, and let innate do its part." It certainly did!

— Doctor of Chiropractic

CASE STUDY

A boy, age 9, diagnosed with Crohn's Disease since the age of 5 came in for chiropractic care after the mother had favorable results for low back pain and sinusitis. This boy was recently placed on daily doses of Flagyl, which seemed to help the severe symptoms somewhat. The patient was placed on an adjustment schedule of 3 times weekly. The patient is now seen once a week, is off all medications and has few attacks of moderate symptoms. Life without fear!

— Doctor of Chiropractic

CASE STUDY

A boy, age 2 1/2, had a prior diagnosis of myoclonic encephelopathy. Symptoms included the child being unable to control body movements. The child was leading a normal, active life until a tuberculin test on November 1, 1989. Within two weeks of the test, the symptoms prevailed. Other symptoms were colic from day 1 and severe sleeping difficulty with onset of myoclonic encephalopathy.

The child was placed under chiropractic care on 04-30-90. We have rendered a total of four adjustments to date with the following areas being adjusted; C1-T9 &L3. The response has been remarkable with the uncontrolled body movements being improved about 80%. The mother and father are astounded with the results. The child at the time of examination was on ACTH and prednisone with negative results. This is typical of success stories in chiropractic offices throughout the country.

— Doctor of Chiropractic

CASE STUDY

Female, age 6, with symptoms including temperatures peaking at 104-105 degrees every day for 2 months. The little girl had been to a large medical center for several evaluations. Complete exams including blood chemistry and UA had been performed. The test results showed no causative factor. Other symptoms were listlessness and constipation. The father contacted me and brought the girl in for chiropractic care. We determined subluxations were present in the atlas and 10th dorsal. An adjustment was made on the first visit. The next day, the father called in and stated that immediately after the adjustment the child's energy level picked up. (The family went to Six Flags and had a great time.) My question to him was, did the temperature go up to 104-105 degrees? He said no, it peaked at 101 degrees and stayed there. The child was adjusted again one week later. Her body temperature normalized and has stayed normal since the 2nd adjustment. Needless to say, the father was elated.

— Doctor of Chiropractic

CASE STUDY

Male, age 10 years old. This was an autistic child with loose bowels and usual autistic symptoms. The chiropractic evaluation revealed subluxations present at occipital C1 and bilateral sacral fixation. The technique utilized in this case was a Right Logan Basic contact. The thermister srip was taped to the patient's back starting at T1 and going to upper midlumbar region. This was tied into a computer which was programmed to measure and record finite temperature changes during the adjusting procedure. A definite heat increase was measured during the adjustment. After 8 adjustments, several symptomatic changes had taken place. The child's teacher remarked that his hyperactive behavior has decreased and that he is able to sit still for 30-40 minutes at a time. His mother also stated that the bowel movements are normal for the first time in many years, and that the child is able to fall asleep easily at night.

— Doctor of Chiropractic

CASE STUDY

Female, 10 months of age. Symptoms include seizures and retardation. The very first seizure occurred at approximately 6 months of age and was very violent in nature. The child was taken to the hospital and was given a strong medication because the seizure was so violent. The side effects of the drug produced brain damage and all normal reflexes disappeared. At 10 months of age, the child was placed under chiropractic care, manifesting a continuous soft cry. After 1 month of care, the cry ceased. In two months, all reflexes reappeared, though overall development was still below normal. The major areas of adjustment were the occipital and atlas. In this case, we utilized a very light thrusting technique. The child was 22 months of age with the physical development of a 1 year old and mental development of 18 months. Her medical pediatrician has since referred other children for chiropractic evaluation due to our success.

— Doctor of Chiropractic

CASE STUDY

Boy, age 11 months. He had severe Downs Syndrome. The boy weighed 7 pounds with no gain since birth. He was unable to retain any nourishment. After the first adjustment, he took 4 ounces of milk. The parents were amazed by this. In the next two weeks, he gained 2 pounds.

— Doctor of Chiropractic

CASE STUDY

Daniel was sitting quietly, which was quite a contrast to his mother, who was nervously pacing the floor. As soon as I sat down, she blurted out, "I heard chiropractors work with children. Daniel's doctors want to put holes inside his gorgeous ears and I won't let them!"

After a few deep breaths, she calmed down enough to say that Daniel had a history of ear infections and for the past year he was having difficulty hearing. His schoolwork went downhill and he began to withdraw from his friends. He got such poor scores on the school hearing test that they suggested putting Daniel into a learning-impaired class. He had been on and off antibiotics since he was a baby and now his pediatricians were suggesting ear tubes.

A chiropractic examination was performed and it was found that two vertebra in his neck were severely misaligned and were pinching the nerves that could affect his ears. Over the next several weeks, he received a series of chiropractic adjustments to realign the bones in his neck. He had no more ear infections, his schoolwork returned to normal and he could stop pretending because he really could hear what his friends were saying.

His hearing was retested at school one year later and it was normal in both ears. His mother was amazed. "Daniel is like a different child. He is no longer withdrawn into himself. He is outgoing and enthusiastic about everything. It's hard to get him to stay still! I haven't stopped thanking my neighbor for insisting I try chiropractic!"

— Doctor of Chiropractic

CASE STUDY

Amanda, at 3 years old, could only have a bowel movement once a week. Her mother said it started a year ago after she fell off a four poster bed. Two adjustments to her lower back and she again returned to her daily bowel habit.

— Doctor of Chiropractic

CASE STUDY

Mary, 7 years old, had such severe asthma that all the doctors in the emergency room knew her by name. Despite all the medication and a completely healthy non-dairy diet, her asthma attacks were still life threatening. Mary started to receive chiropractic care twice a week and within 3 months, Mary is a new child, according to her mother.

"Three months ago, all she could do was sit on the couch and watch television because of her wheezing. Now she runs and roller skates and even plays basketball with her older brother. But the best news of all is she is off all of her medications."

— Doctor of Chiropractic

CASE STUDY

A female at an age of 11 months began chiropractic care as a result of not being able to hold her head up. She also had limited movement on rotation. Three times during this child's late birth, the doctor stated the baby was being carried too low in the birth canal and pushed the head "back up" in the canal. The baby was examined many times with unsuccessful conclusions by the medical doctors.

The parents brought their child in for chiropractic care. The child was x-rayed, which revealed a severe upper cervical problem. The child was adjusted and an immediate response was noted with the child's head moving to the erect position. Both the parents and the grandparents were present during the exam and adjustment and, needless to say, were elated at the result.

— Doctor of Chiropractic

All infants should have their spines checked immediately after entering this world by the chiropractor. Correction of the vertebral subluxation at this time of life means a healthier childhood.

CASE STUDY

Female, age 6. Chief complaints include attention span deficiency, learning disability, lack of bladder control, headaches, sinus infections, constant fever, severely swollen cervical lymph nodes and hyperactivity.

The mother was given morphine during this child's delivery. The mother also received an epidural before the birth. The birth was doctor assisted with the doctor pulling on the head.

The child has taken constant antibiotics since birth. She had tubes put in her ears at 8 months of age. Her body has since rejected them.

She was put under chiropractic care. She was subluxated at the atlas ASL-T9 BR and Sacrum AIR. After 3 months of care, the swollen lymph nodes are now normal, headaches are gone, fevers are gone, no more medications are being taken, and her teachers are now remarking about her being able to concentrate better and her grades have vastly improved. She is now on a maintenance schedule for wellness care.

— Doctor of Chiropractic

CASE STUDY

L.B. is a 63 year old female who came to my office in January of 1997 complaining of radiating pain down her left leg. At the age of seven years (pre-vaccine) she contracted polio. She says she remembers feeling achy all over, had flu-like symptoms, was bed-ridden for two to three weeks, and her right leg went "dead." She was first put into a cast from the right hip to toes and then her right leg was braced for two years. The aftermath of all this medical intervention left her with the following "permanencies." The right side of her body was limp-like, with muscle atrophy of the hip, stomach, thigh and calf on the right side, and loss of balance, speech pathology, ringing in the ears, right foot smaller and loss of hearing. On analysis, thermal and electromyography readings were extremely high. X-rays revealed global subluxation patterns of her entire spine.

Care has been ongoing from January of 1997 through November of 1997, at three times per week. She has received segmental and postural adjustments along with five-point full spine mirror image postural tractioning.

Her response to care has been as follows. Better balance (able to walk on grass and other uneven surfaces), ringing in her ears is gone, hearing is now normal, limp has improved, and speech pathology has not changed. L. B. is astonished at how her body has healed itself. She will continue to receive care three times a week until there is no longer any structural or functional changes in her spine and nervous system. These areas are objectively monitored by x-rays, surface electromyography and thermal scans.

— Doctor of Chiropractic

CASE STUDY

Eleven-and-a-half year old Zoe was brought to my office because of a seizure disorder, chronic ear infections and overall delayed development. On August 12, 1997, Zoe finally came to my office after three prior cancellations of appointments due to her being hospitalized. The history is as follows: birthdate: 9-4-96, birthweight: 6 pounds, 12 ounces, present weight 20 pounds, birth length 21", present length 27". Delivery was two weeks early, the only complications was that it was a forceps delivery. At four to five months, Zoe responded to sound and visual stimulus. Zoe had surgery at the age of 10 days to open her nasal passages (Nasal Atrision). At 11 1/2 months, Zoe could barely hold her head up, it was like getting handed a rag doll, she just flopped over in my hands. She had no grip strength or the ability to close her hands. She could not sit, crawl, or walk. She was in my estimation, developed to about a one to two month old. Zoe has been on maintenance doses of Phenobarbital, Dylantin and even Morphine! Ten to fifteen doses of antibiotics have been given this year, but 23 overall since birth.

Her appetite was poor; she barely ate. Zoe was fed Simlac from day one. Her sleep was always disturbed and she never made it through the night without getting up crying.

Adjustments were given in the cervical spine with a modified activator approach and pediatric diversified adjustments full spine.

On the second visit, the mother reported Zoe made it through the night and slept peacefully since the first visit three days ago. Zoe has made positive progress each and every visit. The mother is telling me of improvements, most of which are obvious measures. She is now sitting almost on her own, holding her head up stronger, using both hands and arms to grasp for things, the grip strength is getting stronger and she is putting the pacifier up to her own mouth.

The appetite is ever increasing. The mother states she has never seen her eat like this. In between visists the mother has stated that Zoe becomes lethargic, but bounces back with more energy after sleep. (I have seen this many times with other children I have cared for.) The grandmother who hasn't seen Zoe in the past month can't believe the difference. After the first week of care the pediatrician, who saw Zoe at least twice a week, called the mother to see where she was and if everything was O.K. Prior to her first visit, over $150,000 had been spent on medical bills.

The one thing I failed to mention up to this point is that Zoe was a twin. Zoe was the weaker of the two. The other twin died two weeks after her first DPT shot at three months of age. Zoe was scheduled for her second DPT shot next week and she will not be present for that shot. The way I see it, chiropractic adjustments have saved this child's life in just the first month of care. I'm going to watch this child grow up!

— Doctor of Chiropractic

CASE STUDY

Marie K. is a 48 year old who sought chiropractic care because of a stiff neck and a painful left knee. She had a skiing accident 20 years ago and never received any treatment or care for the accident. She also had a car accident 10 years ago. She did not experience any symptoms after the accident, but did receive physical therapy.

Marie had a medical history of having depression and panic disorders. She was diagnosed about 1 year ago but has been suffering many years. At the time she presented herself for chiropractic care, she was on an anti-depressant. She explained her concentration and energy level were very low and have been getting worse.

Marie: "Since I have been under chiropractic care, my entire personality has changed. I am more relaxed. Things that used to stress me out no longer do and I treat my husband much better. Our marriage is much better now that I am under chiropractic care. It is truly amazing. I never would have believed it."

"I have also told my friends at the library at which I work. Now they look at me and are amazed how I am able to dance on a knee that gave me so much grief for so long."

"Unexpected side effects from continued care with my chiropractor have been an increase in my overall energy level, improvement in my concentration, and the ability to perform both mentally and physically demanding tasks, such as gardening for long periods of time. My sleeping patterns have improved and my sense of well being. Because of my chiropractor and the adjustments, I feel I am a nicer, more easygoing person to be around. I have a more positive outlook on my life. Because of the rather rapid and dramatic improvement that my husband, neighbors and co-workers saw in me, many of them are now also under chiropractic care."

Marie K. is no longer on her anti-depressant medication and everybody on my staff, as well as other patients, have noticed a tremendous change in her, not only emotionally, but physically as well. As my staff has noticed, she is a "completely different and changed person."

— Doctor of Chiropractic

CASE STUDY

An 88 year old man said, "Doctor, I am an old man. There is nothing left I enjoy doing except reading and I've lost the ability to read. Every time I try to read, my vision blurs out before I read half of a page. I've had three new pairs of glasses in the last six months, but nothing helps. The eye doctor said I'd have to give up reading, but I'd rather die. A friend of mine told me if I came to you, you'll fix it."

I thanked him for the vote of confidence and explained that was not how it worked; that I didn't cure anything. I might, however, remove the impediment and nature might then take care of the problem.

He asked what I thought the problem was and I explained the sub-luxation complex, nerve function and degeneration. After examina-tion, I began his chiropractic care program. I used a modified activa-tor technique and diversified in combination. The day following the 1st adjustment, Mr. P reported he had been able to read 30 minutes but got sleepy and nodded off. "Please explain the problem again," he requested.

I told him that in all probability, the nerve that was involved was one of the ones that regulated blood flow to the eyeball, the optic nerves, and the "seeing centers" of the brain. I explained that there evidently had been enough blood flow to keep the tissue alive but not to allow function when he dropped his head to read. That day he read for two and one half hours as he reported the next day.

On Monday, following the weekend, he showed me he was not wearing either of his hearing aids and stated he could hear better with-out them than he had with them for the last thirty-five years! He asked, "What have you done to me to cause that?" I explained that the same nerve(s) that controlled blood flow to the eyes and seeing mechanism also controlled blood flow to the hearing apparatus and he could have just as easily lost his visual acuity when his hearing went bad.

Neither his original lens prescription, nor any of the later three were correct. He needed less correction to see.

— Doctor of Chiropractic

FAQ - FREQUENTLY ASKED QUESTIONS

Briefly, cover the history of Chiropractic.

The term "Chiropractic" is taken from the Greek, defined as "Done by Hand." Many forms of spinal manipulation have been utilized in healing for thousands of years. The ancient Egyptians, Greeks, American Indians, Chinese and the African cultures have all experimented with spinal manipulation. In the 1800's, medical professionals often used bonesetting as a form of spinal manipulation.

One of the greatest men to recognize the benefit of spinal manipulation was Hippocrates, the Father of Medicine (460 - 377 BC). Hippocrates linked spinal manipulation with ill health. He stated, "get knowledge of the spine, for this is the requisite for many diseases." Hippocrates believed that only nature could heal and it was the physician's duty to remove any obstruction that would prevent the body from healing.

There is a major difference between spinal manipulation and an adjustment. Spinal manipulation is defined as the forceful passive movement of a joint beyond its active limit of motion. It does not imply the use of precision, specificity or the correction of spinal nerve interference. A specific spinal adjustment, on the other hand, is the specific application of forces used to facilitate the body's correction of nerve interference. Chiropractors use specific adjustments to correct nerve interference in your body.

Daniel David (DD) Palmer is considered the "Discoverer of Chiropractic." DD Palmer was born in Port Perry, Ontario, Canada in 1845. In 1865, Palmer moved to the United States. Between 1865 and 1895, he studied health and healing and became a magnetic healer. In 1895, DD made the discovery of chiropractic. This is the date of the first recorded chiropractic spinal adjustment to Mr. Harvey Lillard, who went from being virtually deaf to hearing normal, after DD Palmer delivered a specific and intentional adjustment to his spine.

The most important figure in chiropractic history is definitely, Bartlett Joshua (BJ) Palmer. BJ was only 14 years old when his father discovered chiropractic. However, by 1961, BJ helped elevate chiropractic to the second largest health-care system in America. BJ developed the art, philosophy and science of chiropractic as we know it today. BJ Palmer led the fight along with other chiropractors to practice chiropractic with constant controversy arising from organized medicine. Medical doctors saw chiropractors as a threat because they were taking away many of their patients who were not responding to medicine. This still goes on today. Most medical doctors will not refer patients to a chiropractor.

In the years that followed, the chiropractic profession has grown to include over 60,000 chiropractors in the United States and Canada. Chiropractic schools are graduating approximately 5,000 new chiropractors a year. By the year 2010, it is estimated there will be over 100,000 chiropractors throughout the world.

What type of Education do chiropractors receive?

Chiropractors are very well educated. The science of chiropractic requires doctors of chiropractic to put a special emphasis on anatomy, biomechanics, neurology, pathology, physiology, spinal adjusting techniques, X-ray and related subjects. After intense studies of these subjects, chiropractors are prepared to detect and correct vertebral subluxations, thereby correcting spinal nerve interference.

Number of Classroom Hours Compared to Medical Doctor

Chiropractic		Medicine
540	Anatomy	508
165	Chemistry	325
630	Diagnosis	324
120	Microbiology	114
320	Neurology	112
60	Obstetrics	148
210	Orthopedics	156
360	Pathology	401
240	Physiology	326
60	Psychiatry	144
360	X-ray	148
2,887	**TOTAL HOURS**	**2,706**

In addition to the requirements listed, chiropractors must also complete courses in nutrition, palpation, chiropractic philosophy and practice, and spinal adjustments. Chiropractors have spent 4,485 hours in the classroom, compared to medical doctor's 4, 248 hours, by the time they graduate from chiropractic school. Before they obtain their degree, they must also complete approximately 900 hours of work in a clinic setting.

To graduate with a Doctor of Chiropractic degree, chiropractors must pass a very intense and demanding National Board Examination. In addition, they must also pass a practical exam and interview conducted by the State Board of Chiropractic Examiners in the state where they are seeking a license.

This clearly proves that chiropractors are one of the best trained doctors you will find.

What do Chiropractor's do?

Chiropractors are trained to ensure your nervous system is free of spinal nerve interference. They believe in whole body wellness. Wellness is the state of health where your body is free of spinal nerve interference, allowing you to enjoy life. Your chiropractor will discover any spinal nerve interference within your spinal column and with specific chiropractic adjustments, will correct them. Your body will then be free to heal itself, express itself and function at an optimal level.

Chiropractors teach you how you can live "subluxation-free." This is achieved through better posture, diet, attitude, exercise and rest leading to a higher quality of life.

What are subluxations?

The body depends on the free flow of nerve communication from the brain, through the spinal column, to every part of the body. When any of these nerves become twisted, the vital communication system is interrupted. These neurological interruptions are called subluxations.

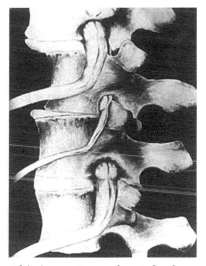

This is one type of vertebral subluxation (spinal nerve interference) — the "silent killer."

What causes vertebral subluxations?

With children, subluxations often occur during the birth process. All of the pulling, pushing and twisting on the newborn's neck and spine during the birth process often cause one or more vertabra to be pushed out of place, resulting in subluxations. As we grow up, subluxations are caused daily by falls, sports activities, accidents/injuries, bad posture, physical and emotional stress and many other things. By having a chiropractor correct these subluxations throughout your childhood and the rest of your life, your family can achieve an improved quality of life.

What are some of the warning signs of subluxations?

Subluxations can cause pain and muscle spasms. However, most of the time, you will not experience any symptoms. Often symptoms such as headaches, back pain, neck stiffness, pain in your shoulders, arms or legs, numbness in your hands and feet and various other symptoms can be signs of subluxations.

How can I try to prevent subluxations?

The number one way to prevent subluxations is to have your chiropractor give you lifetime wellnes care. This way you can come in on a weekly, bi-weekly or monthly basis to get checked.

Other ways to prevent subluxations include proper nutrition, rest, exercise, a positive attitude and good posture. Your body needs healthy foods to replenish itself and repair damage. It is important to exercise to strengthen joints and muscles, so they can support your body's structure. Poor posture can be caused by excessive weight, negative mental attitudes, injury to joints, bones and ligaments, faulty nutrition, improper sleep support, poorly designed shoes and various other contributing factors.

How are subluxations corrected?

Doctors of chiropractic are specifically trained to detect and correct vertebral subluxations. Your chiropractor will perform specific tests, as well as palpation and possibly X-rays, to determine if and where you are subluxated. They will then deliver a specific chiropractic adjustment.

What is a chiropractic adjustment?

A chiropractic adjustment is the art of introducing a specific force in a precise direction, applied to a vertabra that is subluxated. Using the bony processes of the vertebra, it is mostly characterized by a dynamic thrust of controlled amplitude. The adjustment releases the vertebra back into its normal position along the spine, allowing proper nerve flow to and from the brain.

There are numerous ways to adjust the spine. Each of the various techniques require a specific force and line of drive. The adjustment is delivered either by the doctor's hands or a specially designed instrument. Some of the adjusting techniques are quick, while others require a slow constant pressure.

What causes the sound made during a chiropractic adjustment?
The sound is not actually the spine "cracking" or "popping" like most people think. The sound is created by gas rushing in to fill the partial vacuum created when the joints are slightly separated.

Can't I just adjust myself?
No. A chiropractic adjustment is a specific force, applied in a specific direction, to a specific vertebra, and it is impossible to adjust yourself. When you or a friend crack or pop your back and neck, it will give temporary relief, but you have not actually adjusted the subluxation, and it could be very dangerous.

What does it feel like to get adjusted?
Chiropractic patients are very comfortable and relaxed while getting adjusted. An adjustment should not be painful.

Are all patients adjusted the same way?
No. Your chiropractor will take a case history and perform specific chiropractic tests to decide if you are subluxated and what technique they will utilize.
There are numerous techniques taught in chiropractic colleges throughout the world. Your chiropractor is trained in several different techniques and will choose the technique that is best for you.

When should I be adjusted?
Every man, woman and child needs to make an appointment with a chiropractor to have their spine checked on a regular basis. Just like your scheduled dental appointments for proper dental hygiene, you need to have your spine checked on a regular basis.
You should also see a chiropractor if you have any symptoms which make it hard to cope day in and day out. If you have been involved in an accident, you should make an appointment with a doctor of chiropractic.
Remember, chiropractic care is not for the relief of symptoms, conditions or disease. It is essential to correct subluxations, so you continue to function and perform at your highest potential.

Does it hurt to get adjusted?
No. Chiropractic adjustments feel great. When you allow the vertebra in your spine to return to their normal position, there is less stress and tension on your muscles and ligaments.

**Once you get adjusted, do you have to keep
getting adjusted forever?**

No. However, it would be an advantage for you to speak with your chiropractor about lifetime wellness care.

Once your symptoms disappear, you might be tempted to quit care. However, it is important to understand just because your symptoms are gone temporarily, does not mean your spinal problems are corrected. The symptoms are often the first things to disappear. Many spinal subluxations have been neglected since early childhood. These long-standing problems usually involve soft tissue damage, muscle weakness and degenerative changes in the spine. In these cases, ongoing corrective care will help your spine reach optimal health.

If you continue chiropractic care it is ultimately up to you. However, periodic chiropractic check-ups will allow your body to fight off sickness and encourage health.

Is chiropractic care safe?

Yes. Chiropractic care is definitely one of the safest types of health care. Without the use of drugs or surgery, chiropractors utilize a conservative approach when correcting vertebral subluxations. One just needs to compare the malpractice premiums paid by chiropractors to that paid by medical doctors. Chiropractic premiums are approximately 1/20 the price of the premiums medical doctors pay.

Hundreds of thousands of people will die this year as a result of bad medicine. Of the millions of people under chiropractic care, only a handful will even make a complaint.

Can chiropractic help me?

Chiropractic care is beneficial to every man, woman, child and animal that has a spine. Understanding that the brain and spinal cord make up your nervous system, one can understand that chiropractic care works by restoring balance to the body giving it a better chance to heal itself.

Everyone needs proper nerve function. Chiropractic care provides your body with a greater potential to defend itself against germs and infection. You and your family should be checked regularly for spinal nerve interference.

Why do my children need chiropractic care?

The birth process can often be one of the most traumatic events of a child's life. The spine can often be injured during the delivery.

Having your child checked by a chiropractor immediately after birth is a very wise decision. Spinal nerve interference from the birth process often becomes more serious as your child grows up. Only a doctor of chiropractic has the proper training and qualifications to diagnose and correct vertebral subluxations.

Your child's posture is an important indicator of spinal problems. Scoliosis is often caused by improper posture. By having your children checked at a young age, these problems might be prevented.

Children become involved in sports at a young age. These activities can often include minor injuries. When your children play, they are jumping, running, twisting, bumping and falling all over the place. Often they will become subluxated during these activities. To minimize the chance of future health problems it is important to have your children checked by a chiropractor on a regular basis.

Spinal hygiene should be part of your whole family's wellness lifestyle.

Who else needs chiropractic care?

All of your friends should be checked by a chiropractor on a regular basis. Chiropractic care enables your bodies systems to function optimally. You can prevent many future health problems through early detection of vertebral subluxations.

Can I help speed up the healing process?

In a way, yes. Though it is difficult to speed up your body's natural healing process, by following a few recommendations, you can give yourself the opportunity to recover quickly and prevent problems.

It is important that you allow your body enough time to rest throughout the day and when you sleep at night. It is also important to sleep in a proper position. The best way to sleep is on your side with your legs straight and your head on a soft pillow. The next best way is on your back.

When you are lifting objects, always use your legs to lift the weight, not your back. Make sure you are strong enough to lift the object you have in mind. If not, save yourself future injury and ask for help.

It is important to eat a balanced meal. Proper nutrition will provide your body with the essential components for growth and healing.

Try to keep a positive attitude throughout the day and realize life is full of ups and downs. Just when you thought life couldn't get any worse, it won't, it will get better. A positive mental attitude will alleviate stress and allow clear thinking. Stress is known to cause subluxations.

Last, participate in a wellness care program with your chiropractor. Get checked on a regular basis to be the best you can be.

Why should I continue chiropractic care if I do not have symptoms and I feel better?

Chiropractic care is not a treatment or cure for symptoms, conditions or disease. Just because symptoms disappear, doesn't mean your vertebral subluxations are corrected. Many of the cases seen by chiropractors consist of patients who present spinal problems that have developed over many years. Slips, falls, and other accidents experienced over your lifetime adversely affect your spine. The longer you wait to have your spine checked, the longer it will take to correct a problem.

Your chiropractor will suggest a schedule of adjustments to correct your subluxations. Once your body has regained the ability to hold the vertebra in place, you can decide whether you would like to continue with a wellness program.

What typically happens on the first visit?

Typically, on the first visit, you will fill out a complete health history detailing past injuries or problems and present symptoms. Remember, your chiropractor is not asking you about your symptoms because he/she is going to treat them. The symptoms help the chiropractor determine where you are subluxated and what technique to use. Your chiropractor will then review your case history with you and discuss how you may be helped through chiropractic care.

Your chiropractor will then give you a complete examination, consisting of various testing procedures to help determine where you are subluxated.

The chiropractor will then discuss the Report of Findings with you. These are the results of the examination. Your chiropractor will then recommend a specific course of care for you.

How many people are currently seeking care from chiropractors?

Over 25 million people have experienced the remarkable results of chiropractic care. This number continues to grow as more and more people take responsibility for their healthcare and choose noninvasive, drug-free healthcare. Chiropractic care is about one-half the price of medical care.

Glossary

ADJUSTMENT: The specific application of forces used to facilitate the body's correction of nerve interference.

CHIROPRACTIC: A primary health care profession in which professional responsibility and authority are focused on the anatomy of the spine and immediate articulation, and the condition of nerve interference. It is also a practice that encompasses educating, advising about, and addressing nerve interference.

CHIROPRACTIC DIAGNOSIS: A comprehensive process of evaluation of the spinal column and its immediate articulations to determine the presence of nerve interference and other conditions that may contraindicate chiropractic procedures.

CHIROPRACTIC PRACTICE OBJECTIVE: The professional practice objective of chiropractic is to correct nerve interference in a safe, effective manner. The correction is not considered to be a specific cure for any particular symptom or disease. It is applicable to any patient who exhibits nerve interference regardless of the presence or absence of symptoms or disease.

DIS-EASE: The word *disease* is a combination of *dis* and *ease*. *Dis* is a prefix meaning "apart from." It follows then that dis-ease is nothing more than a lack of comfort, a loss of harmony in the system. Chiropractors believe that instead of treating disease with chemicals and invasive procedures, whenever possible, first treat dis-ease with the reduction or elimination of nerve interference, thereby giving the patient a chance to recover naturally before resorting to drugs and surgery.

HEALTH: A state of optimal physical, mental and social well being, not merely the absence of disease or infirmity.

MANIPULATION: The forceful passive movement of a joint beyond its active limit of motion. It doesn't imply the use of precision, specificity or the correction of nerve interference. Therefore, it is not synonymous with chiropractic adjustment.

MEDICAL DIAGNOSIS: Procedures that provide information about disease processes for the selection of treatment.

THE MAJOR PREMISE IN CHIROPRACTIC: A Universal Intelligence is in all matter and continually gives to it all its properties and actions, thus maintaining it in existence.

VITALISM: The doctrine that teaches that in living organisms, life is caused and sustained by a vital principle distinct from all physical and chemical forces. It also teaches that life is, at least in part, self-determining and self-evolving.

VERTEBRAL SUBLUXATION: A misalignment of one or more of the vertebrae in the spinal column, which causes alteration of nerve functions and interference to the transmission of mental impulses resulting in a lessening of the body's Innate ability to express its maximum health potential. Also referred to as nerve interference.

REFERENCES

Chiropractic In New Zealand Report. The Government Printer, Wellington, New Zealand 1979.

Rondberg, Dr. Terry A.: *Chiropractic First.* The Chiropractic Journal, Chandler, AZ 1996.

True Health. World Chiropractic Alliance, Chandler, AZ 1993-1995.

Wardwell, Walter I.: *Chiropractic: History and Evolution of a New Profession,* Mosby Yearbook, St. Louis, MO 1992.

Webster, Dr. Larry L.: *International Chiropractic Pediatric Association.* Stone Mountain, GA 1987-1998.

INDEX